Marilu Henner's
TOTAL HEALTH
MAKEOVER

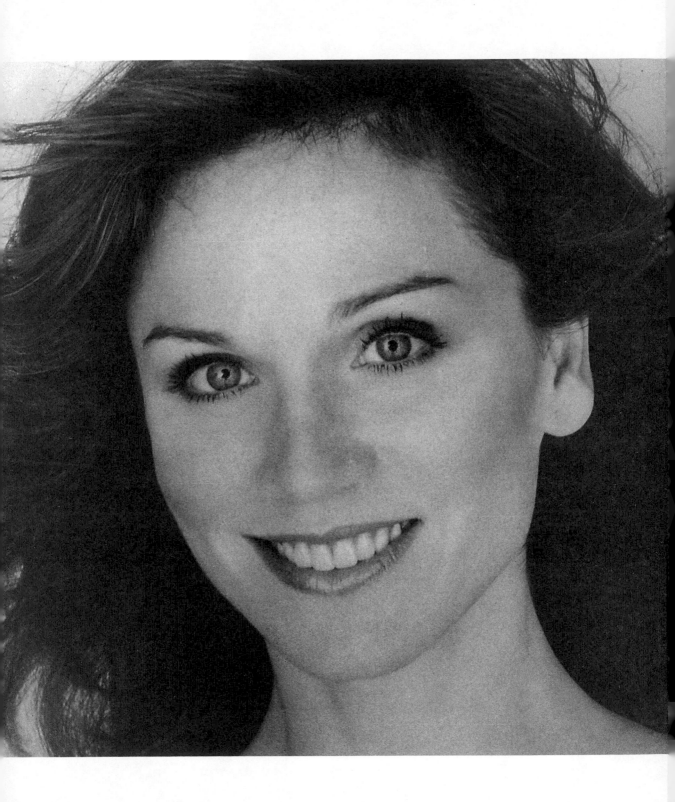

Marilu Henner's
TOTAL HEALTH MAKEOVER

10 Steps to Your B.E.S.T. Body*

* Balance, Energy, Stamina, Toxin-Free

MARILU HENNER
with Laura Morton

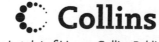
Collins

An Imprint of HarperCollinsPublishers

A hardcover edition of this book was published by HarperCollins Publishers in 1998. A mass-market edition of this book was published in 1999.

MARILU HENNER'S TOTAL HEALTH MAKEOVER. Copyright © 1998 by Marilu Henner. All rights reserved. Printed in the United States of America. No part of this book may be used or reproduced in any manner whatsoever without written permission except in the case of brief quotations embodied in critical articles and reviews. For information address HarperCollins Publishers, 195 Broadway, New York, NY 10007.

HarperCollins books may be purchased for educational, business, or sales promotional use. For information, please e-mail the Special Markets Department at SPsales@harpercollins.com.

FIRST TRADE PAPERBACK EDITION PUBLISHED 2001

Designed by Laura Lindgren

ISBN 0-06-098878-9

16 17 18 ❖/RRD 12 11 10

To my parents,
whose lives and deaths
led me on this road to health.

To Rob, Nicky, and Joey,
who travel the road with me.

Contents

Acknowledgments   xvii

Introduction: Boys and My Weight   xxi

* 1 *

One Step at a Time   1

The Ten Steps—One at a Time   4
What Is Freedom?   9
A Workable Program   10
Excuses, Excuses, Excuses!   12
Marilu's Questions to Think About   13
    Health   13
    Food   13
    Dieting   14
    Body Image   15
What Is B.E.S.T.?   15
"Somewhere over the Rainbow. . ."
    —My Rainbow Theory   16

* 2 *

Balance   19

Understanding Extreme Foods   22
Balance in Your Diet   24
Food and Behavior   26

Changing Your Palate   27

The Art of Chewing   29

Food for Thought   31

    Protein   31

    Carbohydrates   32

    Fat   33

Balancing/Centering Your Body   33

* 3 *
Taking the Plunge   36

Making the Commitment   36

Detoxification and Healing Crises   40

* 4 *
STEP 1: *The Dangers of Chemicals, Additives, and Preservatives*   46

Dangers of Food Additives and Preservatives   49

    Acesulfame K   49

    Artificial Colorings   49

    Aspartame   50

Butylated Hydroxyanisole and Butylated

    Hydroxytoluene (BHA and BHT)   51

    Monosodium Glutamate (MSG)   51

    Nitrites and Nitrates   52

    Olestra   53

    rBGH (Recombinant Bovine Growth Hormone)   54

    Saccharin   54

    Sulfites   54

Organic Food   55

❊ 5 ❊

STEP 2: *Caffeine and Nicotine–* *Breaking the Habit* 58

A Stimulating Brew 58
Caffeine Overload 60
Are You a Java Junkie? 61
Caffeine Health Risks 63
Smoking 65

❊ 6 ❊

STEP 3: *The Not-So-Sweet* *Bad News About* *Sugar and Aspartame* 67

Get off the Sugar Treadmill 69
Sugar Substitutes 71
    Brown Sugar 71
    Saccharin 71
    Aspartame 72
    Acesulfame K 72
    Honey 73
    Sucrose and Fructose 73
    Maltose 73
    Cane Juice 74
    Lactose and Fruit Juice Sweeteners 74
The Scoop on Sugar 76

❋ 7 ❋

STEP 4: *The Health Risks of Meat*   78

Seeing Red—How Animals Are Slaughtered   80
Good Nonmeat Sources of Protein   82

❋ 8 ❋

STEP 5: *The Miracle of Dairy-Free*   84

What's the Matter with Milk?   88
Bovine Slime   94
Dairy and the Cancer Connection   95
Dairy and Nutrient Deficiencies   96
Breast Feeding and Dairy   96
Fat and Dairy Products   98
Dairy Alternatives   101
     Milk   101
     Cheese   102
     Eggs   102
     Butter   103
     Mayonnaise   103
     Ice Cream   103

❋ 9 ❋

STEP 6: *Food Combining— The Winning Combination*   105

Why Food Combining?   106
How Food Combining Works   107

❋ *10* ❋

STEP 7: *Fat—The Good,
the Bad, and the Ugly*   119

The Skinny on Fat   120
Lexicon of Fats   121
Cholesterol   122
Limiting–Not Eliminating–Fat   124

❋ *11* ❋

STEP 8: *The Beauty of
Exercise and Stress Reduction*   127

Stress—What the Hell Is It
   and Why Is It Bugging Me?   134
The Effects of Stress on Your Body   135
Reducing Stress in Your Life   136
   Exercise   138
   Just Say NO!   139
   Laughter Is the Best Medicine   140
   Stress and Eating   141
   Baths and More   142
Skin Brushing—Giving Your Body
   the Big Brush-off   144
How to Skin Brush   145

❋ *12* ❋

STEP 9: *Sleep—The Cure-all*   147

What Is Sleep?   148
The Body's Need to Sleep   149

Contents

Sleep and the Immune System   150
Sleep and the Brain   151
Insomnia   152
    Natural Remedies   154
    To Nap or Not to Nap—That Is the Question 155
Keeping a Sleep Journal   156
Sleep on This   157

* 13 *

STEP 10: *Gusto—*
The Missing Ingredient
in the Mind/Body Connection   158

Are You Ready for Gusto?   160
    My "Toy Box" Theory   161
    Looking Good, Feeling Good   162
Confidence and Self-Esteem   164
Gusto and Food   165
Setting Goals—A Road Map to Gusto   166
Imagery and Visualization   167

* 14 *

Why Certain Diets Work
and Others Don't   168

Die-it   168
Live-it   171
Diet Roulette   172
Men Versus Women   174
    Childhood Eating Habits   174
    Overweight Men and Women   176

The No-Fat Explosion   178
Is There a Magic Pill?   180
What Is Obese?   181
Finding Your Ideal Weight   183
Readjusting Your Weight Set Point   184

* 15 *
Is Heredity Destiny?
To See Your Future,
You Must Know Your Past   185

Is Heredity Destiny?   186
Understanding Your Genes   190
   Obesity   191
   High Blood Pressure   191
   Heart Disease   192
   Depression   193
   Cancer   195
   Osteoporosis   195
   Diabetes   198

* 16 *
Reading Your Face   200

How to Read Your Face   201
Getting Under Your Skin   204
Vitamins and Minerals That Help
   Your Complexion   207

* 17 *
What's the Poop?   209

Your Digestive System and How it Works   210
The Poop on Poop   213
  Frequency of Elimination   213
  Stool Weight   214
  Transit Time   215
  Stool Consistency   215
  Effort   216
Digestive Disorders   217
  Gas   218
  Constipation   220
  Diarrhea   222
  Irritable Bowel Syndrome/Inflammatory
    Bowel Disease   224
  Heartburn   227
Fix It with Fiber   228

* 18 *
Listening to Your Body   232

How to Set Up and Keep a Lifestyle Journal   235
Tracking Your Weight   236
  What to Put in Your Journal   236
Tracking Your Food   237
Food Allergies and Food Intolerances   238
  What to Put in Your Journal   241
Tracking Your Exercise   241
  What to Put in Your Journal   241
Tracking Your Bathroom Activity   242
  What to Put in Your Journal   242

Contents

Tracking Your Sleep   242
    What to Put in Your Journal   242
Tracking Your Menstrual Cycle   243
    What to Put in Your Journal   243

✻ 19 ✻
Alternative/Preventive Medicine   245

East Versus West   247
Alternative Medicines and Treatments:
    Do They Work?   248
        Acupuncture   248
        Shiatsu and Acupressure   249
        Homeopathic Medicine   249
        Herbs/Supplements   251
Marilu's Secret Cure-alls   253
        Cold Sores   253
        Colds   253
        Headaches   254
        Jet Lag   254
        Morning Sickness   254
        Motion Sickness   255
        PMS   255
        Sprains   255

✻ 20 ✻
Practical Living in Your New
Total Health Makeover World   256

How to Order in a Restaurant   257
        T.G.I.Friday's   261
        Chinese Restaurant   261

Josie's   262
Deli   262
Italian Restaurant   263
Stocking Your Pantry   264
Breakfast Items   264
Lunch and Dinner Items   265
Snacks   265
Cheese Substitutes   266
Condiments   266
Drinks   267
Eating at a Friend's Home   268
Flying   269
Marilu Henner 101   270
Things I Have Learned About Health   270
Things I Have Learned About Food   270
Beauty Tips   271
Things I Have Learned from Macrobiotics   272
Things I Have Learned from My Parents   272
Things My Therapist Says   272
Things My Life Has Taught Me   272
Things I Say to My Kids   274
Things My Kids Say   274
B.E.S.T. Advice   274

* 21 *

Some Final Thoughts

Some Final Thoughts   275

Appendix A: Rich Sources of Nutrients   277
Appendix B: Josie's Recipes   283
Bibliography   307
Index   311

Acknowledgments

This book is the brainchild of the inimitable Judith Regan, who for the six years of our friendship has picked my brain for my latest and greatest discovery about healthy living, and has called me for natural remedies whenever something was wrong with her or her kids. Finally, she said, "Why don't you just write a book about all of this stuff?" Her vision, her encouragement, her professionalism, her taste, her quick thinking, and her talent for knowing what works make her my idol.

Her fabulous and dedicated team at ReganBooks and Harper-Collins, John Ekizian, Jennifer Nicolosi, Steven Sorrentino, Paul Olsewsky, Dana Isaacson, Angelica Canales, Joseph Rutt, Linda Dingler, Patricia Wolf, Laura Lindgren, and John Day, all worked so hard to get this book out on time. Thank you!

To my *Chicago* buddies, who let me teach them about the evils of dairy and sugar between shows and who showed me their gusto about eating birthday cakes between acts: Jimmy Borstelmann, Marcia Lewis, Lillie Kae Stevens, Paula Davis, Jo-Ann Bethell, Terry Whitter, Michael Berresse, Todd Heughen, Mindy Farbrother, Steven Keough, Leigh Zimmerman, Ernie Sabella. A special thank you to Pete Sanders, Helene Davis, and Clint Bond Jr. for their help with photographs, and an extra special thank you to Barry and Fran Weisler, the wonderful producers of *Chicago*.

To the people who make up the team roster of my life, no matter what project I'm on: my William Morris agents Mel Berger and Dan Strone, Marc Schwartz and his assistant John Gill; my publicist Dick Guttman and his assistant Susan Madore; the dynamic duo of Provident Financial Management, Richard Feldstein and Barbara Karrol; my teacher and number one doctor for the last nineteen years, the gifted and knowledgeable Dr. Thich

AnThanh; and last, but certainly not ever least, the brilliant and incomparable Dr. Ruth Velikovsky Sharon.

To my friends who contributed to this book with either their words or their photographs, Fran Drescher, John Matoian, Michael Caine, MaryAnn Hennings, Maggie Gillott Fountain, Dan LaMorte, Tom Moore, Michael Lembeck, and Dr. Belvedere. Thank you for your contributions and friendship.

To my family, whose love and support have guided me throughout my life, and who have put up with all my experimentation and zealousness (and I told you so's!), Christal Henner and Roy Welland, Tom and Dr. Melody Alderman, Lynnette Lesko Henner, Elizabeth Carney, Suzanne Carney, Erin Lieberman, Lorne Lieberman, Sally Lieberman, Bill Drake, and especially JoAnn Carney and Tom Henner for all their help with photographs. A very special thank you to Donna Erickson, without whom I couldn't do half the things I do. Knowing that my children are in such good hands when I'm not there is greatly reassuring to me.

The writing of this book could never have been accomplished without the hard work, unquenchable team spirit, and necessary sense of humor of the amazing group of people who came together to turn my vision into a reality. Jim Sperber and Danielle Caiet-Bordwin, who collectively handled all the coordination of the photographs and many other essential elements that make up the essence of this book. They came in every day with a get-it-done spirit and an eventual nonsugar, nondairy smile. Debbie Babroski, for all of her terrific research and for being such a whiz on the computer. Louis Lanza, who supplied us with the recipes for some of the greatest food I've ever eaten, not to mention a few late-night snacks. Tom Eckerle, whose photographs make great food look their B.E.S.T.! Mindy Herman, RD, who helped to prove the recipes are really healthy; Elena Lewis, who rummaged through all my photographs long distance, and made sure they got to me on time and in good shape. My brother, Lorin Henner, who once again added his special sense of humor and unflappable support. And to Laura Morton, whose patience, positivism, resilience, organization, apartment, social contacts, menu folder, writing talent minus spelling ability, work-in-progress sense of humor, comfortable desk area, and the healthiest ego in town provided the motor for this project as well as some of the best laughs and good feelings you can share with someone, especially under such intense time constraints. You're the best!

Thank you, team, I love you all!

Finally, to my loving husband, Rob, who once again has understood the pressures and commitment to an enormous project and never complained, only supported. It's wonderful to be in love with someone who lets you be who you are. And to my two boys, Nicky and Joey, who not only provide me with the two best reasons for being healthy, but also give me the greatest joy I've ever known.

Introduction

BOYS AND MY WEIGHT

The question I've been asked most often over the last ten years is, "Marilu, why are you much thinner now and even younger-looking than you were when you did *Taxi* in the seventies?" Well, I know that people are being kind and they ask this to make me feel good, but I also know that there is a lot of truth to it. I am much thinner than I was. I have much more energy. I really feel great. And yes, I do think I look much better. As far as younger-looking, well, I don't know about that, but I do know that I *feel* much younger than I did even in my twenties, and I'm forty-five. Except for during my pregnancies, my weight has not fluctuated more than five pounds in the last eleven years. So this is not a temporary phase I'm going through.

So how did all this happen? What changed my weight, my looks, my energy, and ultimately my life? A diet? Pills? Liposuction? Cosmetic surgery? *No, no, no, and ABSOLUTELY not!* Do I eat every day like a gerbil or a bird? Do I spend six hours a day working out? Again, no and no. After nineteen years of experimenting, a thousand mistakes, over 400 books (read, not written), at least 200 bad diets over my lifetime, five doctors, four physical therapists, three nutritionists, two personal trainers, one therapist, and a partridge in a pear tree, I have found what I believe are the best answers this planet (both hemispheres, East and West) has to offer about living a happy, healthy, and balanced life.

If I didn't take care of myself the way I do, I could never be living the life I am living now. I'm a wife, a mother, an actress, and an author. While writing this book, I have been performing in the

Broadway show *Chicago* (eight performances a week), as well as being a mom to my beautiful sons, Nicky (age 3½) and Joey (age 2).

My program, lifestyle, philosophy, or whatever you want to call it, has been working beautifully for my family and me for the last eleven years. I have become sort of a Pied Piper of healthy living for my friends as well. My Total Health Makeover is now working for at least a hundred of my friends, too. Most of them claim to have converted followers of their own. (Just like that old shampoo commercial, where you tell two friends and they tell two friends, and so on, and so on . . .) It's easy to find converts, because once they question my program, learn about it, apply it, and see the results, they know it works and continue to follow it.

From the very first page of this book, I want you to know that **I love food**. I am truly a girl who loves to eat. There's something luscious and gratifying about food. Its smells, its tastes, its textures can drive me crazy. My fondest memories from my childhood as well as adulthood are all centered around some great meal. Bringing a group together and enjoying the social interaction of being with people who are laughing and smiling and feeling full of life gives me such joy. I adore going out with my family and friends, eating and drinking, and having a wonderful time. Over the years, after trying every crazy diet known to man, I realized that I could not and would not allow myself to be controlled by food and live a life of deprivation. I needed to be actively living a lifestyle that made food my friend and not my enemy. It took nineteen years of learning how to balance the relationship between healthy eating habits and my passion for food. Actually, it took me eight years to figure it out and eleven years of practice and perfecting this connection. But I've succeeded and have lived a truly healthy life since 1987. I've had my ups and downs over the years (and I mean in every area of my life—from my weight, to my career, to my personal relationships). But finding balance has made it easier for me to ride the roller coaster. Today, I have a beautiful family and many joyous blessings to celebrate, and I want to share my personal discoveries with you. Maybe you'll be able to relate to the information, and I hope you'll make some positive changes in your life that help you realize the life you were born to live. Our time on this planet is far too short not to be our best. Change is never easy, but it is an ever-present aspect to growth and self-improvement. It takes only one person to change your life, and that is you.

Writing this book has been a lot of fun for me. Having the opportunity to relive so many experiences and share them with you is the best way I can think of to inspire and motivate you. I've been through a lot over the years, and my experiences and experiments with food and dieting are the inspiration for writing this book. My program described within these pages is not just about diet, though. It's a Total Health Makeover. It's an adaptation in lifestyle designed to reprogram the way you think and feel about your health and your body, whether you're fat or thin.

When my parents both died in their fifties (my father at fifty-two from a heart attack, and my mother at fifty-eight from arthritis complications), I was devastated. At the time, I didn't fully understand that changing their eating and health habits could have prevented or at least alleviated some of their health problems. But now, after nineteen years of research and personal practice, I have created the healthiest, easiest program to make yourself over and to create the best *you* ever. It's a program that I have developed over the years that works for me. Think of me as your personal guide and this book as your "Cliff's Notes" to becoming a happier, healthier you. The key is finding your balance.

I wanted to call my first book *Boys and My Weight* because every pivotal moment and every event of my life can be measured in some way by my relationships . . . both with men *and* with food. I can tell you how much I weighed at any point in my life from the summer between eighth grade and high school (my boyfriend was Steve and I weighed 125 pounds) through college (my boyfriends were Jim, Tom, and Doug and I weighed 155–160). I remember how much I weighed during every episode of *Taxi* (the range was 127–142, and I dated, married, and divorced my first husband at the time, though there were a few cast members along the way . . . not to mention John Travolta!). Today, I am happily married (for eight years) to my husband, Rob, and I'm still totally aware of my current weight fluctuations (119–124). In the past, I would mark my birthdays by whom I was dating and how much I weighed. I guess that's why you could call this a running theme in my life . . . boys and my weight.

I grew up in a typical Midwestern family. Meals weren't complete unless they had one representative from each of the major food groups, especially meat. It's funny when I look back on my childhood from my perspective today and consider the foods I liked and didn't like. I loved sugar. I was completely addicted to it, as are most children. I would put sugar on everything, my Frosted Flakes, my Sugar Pops, even my toast! After school, I'd shop for my mother at the local grocery store and spend my "money for going" on candy. As a twelve-year-old baby-sitter, I would eat the parents out of house and home. Especially cookies and chips. My deal was 50 cents an hour and all I could eat.

I wasn't much of a milk drinker. I just didn't like it. In those days, everyone, even the nuns at school, tried to convince me to "drink my milk." That sure never stopped me from immensely enjoying other dairy products like cheese and ice cream, though my favorite cheese was American cheese, which of course meant that I really had a thing for processed food. Processed food, which isn't even "real" food, simply tasted better to me at the time. Salty processed cheese and refined sugar were my two favorite foods. That's how destroyed my palate was at twelve years old.

Becoming aware of my own body and self-image at a fairly early age helped me develop, and in many ways *destroyed* my metabolism for years to come. I remember being thirteen and in the eighth grade. Typical of that age, I hung around with a bunch of girls whose main topics of conversation were (you guessed it) boys and our weight.

I always felt athletic and in pretty good shape as a kid. My family owned a dancing school, and I took lessons my whole childhood. But as any thirteen-year-old will tell you, it's not easy to escape peer pressure. I wanted to look good for the big school dance, so maybe I'd skip dinner one night. I would convince myself that if I ate only French fries after school and skipped my dinner, it would be smarter than eating both. In remembering these stories, I unearthed my diary from that year of my life, and I thought you might find it amusing, as I sure did, to see some of those eighth-grade entries. See if these spark any similar memories for you . . .

Thursday, June 16, 1966

I feel so fat and ugly today. I ate way too much at the picnic on Monday. Oh why oh why do I do things like that? I hate myself today. I really want to look good for the teen club dance tomorrow night. Maybe if I don't eat dinner, then maybe Donny will notice me tomorrow.

Friday, June 17, 1966

HE NOTICED ME! I looked so cute in my loden green and white striped poor boy and matching loden green skirt. All the girls were jealous, especially that Diane. I know she likes Donny as much as I do, but HA! HA! He danced with me. Twice! (And one of them was even slow.) I feel happier, thinner, and more beautiful.

P.S. Terry watched me from the window and Steve said he wanted to walk me home. Holy Confusion! What am I going to do???? Thank you God for letting sooo many boys like me.

I got into the mentality of dieting, and I bought my first calorie-counting book. I remember that book describing the ideal portion size as the size of a deck of playing cards. That was equal to almost four ounces of meat, which was the recommended portion in those days. How ridiculous to be thinking about portion size at age fourteen, but think about it I did, and so I was always measuring things and counting calories, and you know what happened? *I started to gain weight.* In the past, I pretty much ate when I was hungry, and because I was always so physically active, I evenly maintained my weight. I was getting plenty of exercise whether I was dancing or running around the neighborhood playing with my friends. But as soon as I started obsessing over what I ate, how much I ate, when I ate, and then fasting and pigging out, it defied my natural appetite. I was meticulous about what I put into my mouth and ever so careful not to exceed that 1,200-calorie-a-day allowance I gave myself. Needless to say, my eating habits, let alone my metabolism, were changed—no, make that screwed up—for the next twenty years.

When I entered high school I really started to experiment with every cockamamie crazy diet known to man . . . and even a few of my own yet unknown, too! Let's see, there was the "ice cream diet" where you eat half a gallon of vanilla ice cream a day for three days. It supposedly dehydrates you, and you'll apparently lose lots of weight. It didn't work (and in fact all it did was constipate me), but it made so much sense in the tenth grade. I tried the "graham cracker and peanut butter diet," where you eat a spoonful of peanut butter on a graham cracker every two hours. I went on the "Stillman diet," eating only protein, like bacon and fried eggs or a cheese omelet. There were limited carbohydrates on the diet, so after a week of protein only, I was carbohydrate-starved. I ended up stuffing myself with whatever carbohydrates I could get my hands on, like cookies or chips. Then there was the "starvation diet." In fact, I remember making it ten days on the starvation diet before I broke it by eating a baked Alaska. The second time I went on the starvation diet, I made it five days until I gave in to an UNO's pizza. I even came up with my "if it isn't in the calorie-counting book it has no calories diet"! Okay, so I'll admit that even then I knew I was pushing the envelope a bit on this one, but how many calories could an orange rind have, anyway? I absolutely could not find any solid evidence of an orange rind having any calories anywhere, so therefore, it *must* have no calories!

You name it, I tried it, and usually with little or no success. But that was so typical for me. It was either feast or famine. I ate at such extremes, and my diet was always out of balance.

Throughout high school I continued this whole yo-yo mentality of dieting and losing weight, which was often set off by the need to lose weight especially for a particular event. Unfortunately, I became absolutely fixated and certain that everything I would ever do in my life would be determined by how much I weighed. I became obsessed with reading those body weight charts put out by insurance companies to see if I fell within their guidelines. I would look at myself in the mirror and think I looked obese when I was totally foxed out and dressed up. Psychologically, I couldn't accurately see the reflection in the mirror anymore. I had absolutely no concept of proper nutrition, let alone any real connection to how I looked, and this went on for years. In fact, I started to play a mind game with myself; I would set the scale back ten pounds so that when I weighed myself I wouldn't have to see my "real" weight. I have always been a whiz at numbers, so calculating the weight was never a problem. I just couldn't face the idea of stepping on a scale and reading my actual weight, no matter what it was. I finally had to break this habit when digital scales came along, and I no longer could lower the weight. So much for the virtues of progress and the digital age!

My weight wasn't my only teenage battle. I ate a lot of candy and greasy foods as a teenager, so I constantly dealt with breakouts. I knew certain foods had a reputation for making you break out, but I never made a connection to them at the time. I ate French fries and cheeseburgers. I liked junk food, especially candy, but how could I know at fourteen that my eating habits were the cause of my zits *and* my constipation?

The summer between high school and college, I went off to work at a resort in Wisconsin, and literally worked and ate like a horse. I was not a happy camper that summer, and I guess my emotions manifested themselves as out-of-control eating habits. I was mourning the loss of my father the previous Christmas, and I just was not feeling good about myself. My boyfriend at the time, Steve, came along, and I wasn't even nice to him. I was in a total funk. I wish I had known then what I know now about weight control, because instead of gorging myself that summer I could have made my resort experience like going to a spa. Everything I needed, food- and activity-wise, was available to me, but I didn't have a clue. When I came home, everyone was shocked, to say the least, because I had gained so much weight. When I stepped on that scale at home, even though I lowered it by the usual ten pounds, I just about died. I had gained twenty-five pounds in seven weeks.

I always had the ability to figure out some plan to take off the pounds when I put them on, but this time it was going to be extra hard work. What I hadn't mastered yet was redefining my relationship with food. I didn't realize I would stay on the weight-gain-and-weight-loss roller coaster until I figured it out. The whole yo-yo mentality of dieting is so unhealthy, and yet so many people have it. We even watch famous role models go through the dieting turmoil. No matter who you are, you'll always end up gaining that weight back times two if you don't shed the excess weight in a healthy manner.

After that summer, I started my freshman year at the University of Chicago, and I remember being totally humiliated because during a required medical examination they made you weigh in before you could start classes. I had been dieting, but I certainly hadn't lost all the weight I wanted to yet. I had maybe lost ten pounds, and the thought of getting on that scale was more than I could bear. I can actually remember the school nurse saying out loud, "Oh, we'll have to move this up a notch" when I finally did step on the scale. I just wanted to smack her, and I definitely wanted to stop her hand from sliding that chrome plate up to the next notch, which was the 150-pound mark, and then some.

I was wearing Levi's that were size 34 x 34, and I thought they looked really cool on me because they were a little bit long and I guess I was under the impression they elongated my body. I'd wear really high boots to give myself a long, lean-leg look, and camou-flage myself behind big men's-styled shirts. It was hilarious, but at the time, I just figured that if I were frenetic and moved around a lot, no one could stare at me long enough to really see what I looked like. How could anyone focus in on a constantly moving target? In my mind, this was a perfect solution so that no one could possibly notice that I was a little "chubby." People used to whisper behind my back, "You should have seen her a few years ago. She was really hot." How could I have peaked at age sixteen? No way! This wasn't happening to me. And yet, despite my pants size, I always had a big personality to compensate, so socially speaking, I was rarely without a date.

My sophomore and junior years of college were more of the same up-and-down struggle, until one day I got a call from an old friend, Jim Jacobs. We had worked together on *Grease*, the show he had written when I was a freshman and he had since taken the show to Broadway. They were getting ready to cast for the National Touring Company, and Jim called to ask me to come to New York and audition. After a moment of hesitation, I was on a plane and auditioning for the producers and choreographer. They asked me to hang around and grab a coffee at the coffee shop next door to the theater, and I remember thinking to myself how badly I wanted this job. The good news is I got the part, and the bad news? They wanted me to lose weight. Oh yeah . . . no problem . . . They never told me by when . . .

I was on the road in *Grease*, and to this day I can tell you which city we were in by how good the food was. I know the best cheese shops in Pittsburgh, and that the best Reuben sandwich you'll ever have can be found in Cleveland. We would eat huge pots of fondue and giant butterscotch sundaes. This was some diet I was on. I was always eating something greasy, fatty, and cheesy. I was taking the title of the show to extremes by living it in my diet! One night, the cast and I were out to dinner, and some people came over to our table to say hello. They were trying to guess who was playing which part, and Barry Bostwick, the hunky star of the Broadway

Co., points to me and says, "Obviously, you're Cha-Cha, right"? Cha-Cha was then the fat girl in the show and I had been cast as Marty, the bombshell! I couldn't believe that my idol thought I was playing the fat girl, except in retrospect, I could have and probably should have been, because that's exactly what I was.

I always had relatively thin legs, so I could get away with squeezing into a size 14 dress and still look pretty good. I just looked voluptuous. I would see myself in photographs standing next to other people and convince myself that the camera angle was simply unflattering. It never dawned on me that I might actually be heavy. I totally convinced myself at the time that I was getting away with this charade. I was on a diet for a solid three weeks, losing about ten pounds, and when I got on the scale I was certain I would be less than 140 pounds. It was my twenty-first birthday, and as a present to myself, I wanted to lose that weight. To my horror, when I stepped on that scale, it said 160! Something had to give, and it wasn't going to be my seams.

When I went home to Chicago later that summer of my twenty-first year, the real bomb was about to drop. Several friends and family members came to see me perform, including a family I used to baby-sit for when I was younger. The father came backstage after the show and said something to me I will never forget. He said, "Marilu, you are so talented. And as someone who loves you, I am telling you that if you want to be successful in this business, you must lose some weight. You deserve to have a big career, and you're not going to have it unless you drop twenty-five to thirty pounds." These were words only a father could say with love, and had my dad still been alive, I am certain he would have said those very same words to me that day. Believe me, those loving words of advice changed my life forever.

The very next day I went to two fellow cast members who had recently lost weight, and I asked them for their help. One of the guys had lost a lot of weight quickly on a particular diet, so I followed his lead and went on that program and triumphantly shed twenty pounds in two months. This was the first time that I felt somewhat balanced while dieting. I became very intrigued by the food I was consuming. I wanted to understand every fiber that made up the chemical composition of each morsel. I wanted to grasp what an apple was—I mean what it really is made up of. I started to write down everything and measure my portions. This was the beginning of learning a new relationship with food.

I had lost twenty-three pounds, and was feeling really great about how I looked. In December I went to New York to visit a girlfriend of mine who had also been in *Grease*. I walked into the theater, and no one recognized me. They had never seen me weigh so little since I had started in the national tour, and I was definitely a fraction of who I had been. The producers had asked me to sing a number for them for their new show, and I happily obliged. A week later, I was asked to come back to New York for a final audition for the Broadway company of *Over Here*. The next day, I had the job. I was Broadway bound! And I guess you could say that if I hadn't heeded the advice of a loving friend, I would probably never have lost that weight. Clearly, those extra pounds were weighing me down far more than in weight. The weight was like an iron ball and chain imprisoning me from my destiny. It was holding me back from a future filled with happiness, health, and success.

I saw my mother healthy for the last time during Christmas 1977. I had moved to California to pursue my career, and went back home to Chicago to see her the following April. I wasn't prepared at all for this vision of a woman who vaguely resembled my mom. My family had seen her on a fairly regular basis so I guess they didn't recognize just how frail she had become, and I certainly had no warning before I walked into her hospital room. As I spent time with her, I could see how hard her body was working to try to heal itself, but her strength was depleted. My mother had gone from teaching dancing in December, to getting the flu in January, to being hospitalized in February, to having her leg amputated in April. She died in May. Her body just shut down until finally she passed away. How could something like this happen? The doctors had no real explanation for the total breakdown of my mother's health, and yet, she was gone. I remember thinking that we had lost our father at fifty-two from a heart attack, and now our mother at fifty-eight of complications from arthritis! Is this what my brothers, sisters, and I had to look forward to?

Our bodies are well-made machines, and if we treat them properly, they should not break down prematurely. I made up my mind that day I was not going to let my mother's death be in vain. This would not happen to me or to anyone else in my family. Two weeks after my mother's death, I began reading voraciously about food and its connection to health. I started to study alternative health practices and ideas that have since influenced how I live my life.

Well, the rest of my story unfolds its wings throughout the following pages of this book. This is my story of finding my road to health and overcoming the hurdles and pitfalls of everyday life. I've been up and I've been down. I have tried and triumphed, and I have also failed. I am as human as you are. My good fortune of becoming an actress has granted me many perks in life, but they sure haven't given me a ticket to bypass life's roadblocks. I might be able to get you good tickets to a Broadway show these days, but there is no such thing as a good ticket broker for this thing called your life. Untangle the web that you have woven for yourself, and you may find that you have the ability to be the star of your own show. You may discover your own road to health and happiness . . . and to your life.

The key to unlock that door lies within these pages. Read on and enjoy the journey. . .

1 | One Step at a Time

APPROXIMATELY 400,000 AMERICANS A YEAR DIE
AS A RESULT OF AN UNHEALTHY DIET AND A
SEDENTARY LIFESTYLE.

Now that I've got your attention: *When was the last time you felt healthy?* Do you think you feel healthy right now . . . this very instant? Look around you. Take a look at who you see walking around the shopping mall or in line at the movie theater. What do you see when you're at an airport? Do these people look healthy to you? Really take a good look around, and I think you'll be hard-pressed to find a truly vibrant, healthy person, someone who has skin that's tight and smooth, alert eyes, positive mental energy, and a look of real physical fitness. As human beings, we have taken ourselves so far away from our natural instincts. We don't walk with good posture, we carry excess baggage (physical and emotional) like it was designer luggage. We eat completely unnatural foods for our bodies, and basically live a very different lifestyle from the one we were intended to live. When I watch the Discovery Channel with my kids, I'm always so respectful of how animals eat and live the way nature intended. You never see a giraffe with a spare tire or a panther with cellulite. When I look around, I'm struck by how much less healthy human animals look compared with the animals I see on TV. And believe me, I'm not saying that we should all be naked, in fact far from that. (Would you want to see most of the people you see in a mall with their clothes off?)

It's time to wake up and realize that on the whole, even if you *think* you feel healthy and strong, you probably don't. The problem with knowing how you're feeling is identifying what "healthy" feels like. How do you look to everyone else? Most people walk around a little slouched over, completely stressed out, and at least slightly overweight. We're not even staying the same shape that human beings were intended to be. As we gain weight, we actually distort our natural body outline and become a misshapen version of the human form. If you are nodding your head in agreement right now, you are the perfect candidate for my program. Do you have the guts to read on?

As a society, Americans eat a higher-fat diet than people in most other cultures, and we live a life of fast food and instant meals. Who has the time to cook anymore? From a health perspective, we don't take care of ourselves as we should. We ignore common ailments, put off that workout, completely overwork ourselves, and underestimate our need for sleep. Do any of these sound familiar? Then it is time to make a change in your life! We know so much more now than we ever have before about health and diet. I believe that many people are ready to make that change and are finally willing to take the right steps toward becoming healthy.

Most of us are very trusting people and believe what we're told and everything we read. We really buy into the idea that if something is available and we're told it's good for us, it must be okay, yet we never look beyond that. The truth is, we're manipulated by the media and by food manufacturers. There's so much conflicting information out there, how can you possibly know whom to believe? Should we be eating a high-protein, low-carbohydrate diet, or is it a high-fiber, low-protein diet? Does fat-free mean it's good for you? It's all so confusing. We certainly don't take the time to read food labels as we should. I mean, if you can't pronounce it, why in the world would you put it in your body? Anything with a food label that reads, "Continued on the next can" should not be a part of your regular eating habits. It's a good indication that it's not a "real" food for your "real" body. We have to educate ourselves so that we can make a move to take that first step. That's why I have created this easy-to-understand ten-step program.

The plan in this book is a simple one, but it has the power to bring your health and vitality to a new level, and add years to your life. My ten-step program is really about liberating yourself from your old habits. It frees you from learned behavior. Once you discover that you have a choice about what you eat and how you live your life, you will find that my program is the opposite of deprivation. It is, in fact, a path to freedom. Take this information and process it as if you were a computer updating an old program. It takes a little while to load in the information, but the upgrade is definitely worth it. Suddenly, your computer can do things it never could before. It's faster and more productive. The upgrade just makes your life easier. Sounds good, doesn't it?

Ask yourself one question. Am I the best version of myself? Most of you may not even be able to answer that question honestly at this moment. You may not know the truth. Can you handle the truth? Well, I am certain that by virtue of your having gone out and bought my book, you must be on a quest for a better life. If that is your goal, read on.

What are the ten steps? They're ten things that, over the years, and through much investigation and experimentation, I changed about my life. I knew that I wanted to get healthy and feel great, but I didn't want it to be a temporary change. I created a lifestyle that worked for me, and if you follow just one of these steps, you'll definitely feel better. If you follow more than one, you'll feel better than you ever have. And if you follow all ten steps you'll be your B.E.S.T. The overall idea is to reexamine your relationship with food, your lifestyle, and your health. Pick any one step and decide if you want to try the beginner, intermediate, or advanced version of that step. Try the version you've chosen for at least three weeks to feel a difference. If you don't feel a difference after one week, you may be ready for the next level. If after three weeks the advanced version of the step you took doesn't create a significant change in your life, and you decide to go back to your old ways, at least you'll always know the B.E.S.T. way to live. Try to enjoy the process. It will make the changes you experience that much easier to handle and accept. And by the way, don't get obsessed over your makeover. It's been designed to be a step-by-step process. Otherwise, you'll become what I call a "makeover maniac."

The Ten Steps—One at a Time

1. CHEMICALS

BEGINNER. Continue eating the way you have been, but now read every label on every can, box, or bag of food you eat to become aware of all the chemicals that enter your body daily. You're not changing your diet, you're only changing your *awareness*.

INTERMEDIATE. Same as beginner, plus try to eliminate all those products that *barely resemble* real food. Anything that takes an entire paragraph to describe its ingredients is a good place to start.

ADVANCED. Try to eliminate all foods that contain harmful chemicals, and make nonchemical real foods the majority of your diet.

MAKEOVER MANIAC. Fill a knapsack with organic brown rice, shave your head, and move to Tibet.

2. CAFFEINE

BEGINNER. No more than two caffeine beverages a day (two cups of coffee, or one coffee and one tea, etc.). Remember, I'm talking about a normal six-ounce beverage. No triple espresso super-grande bucket-o'-caffeine specials.

INTERMEDIATE. No more than five caffeine foods or beverages a week.

ADVANCED. Try to eliminate caffeine from your diet. This includes coffee, tea, most soft drinks, and chocolate.

MAKEOVER MANIAC. Become an anticaffeine activist. Splash buckets of coffee bean vine sap on patrons at Starbucks.

3. SUGAR

BEGINNER. Each day, allow yourself two *added* teaspoons of sugar, preferably in the raw. (Not you silly, the sugar!) Continue to allow yourself the sugar that's already in the food you eat, but (and this is very important) *be aware* of the amounts in each food (e.g., there are ten teaspoons of sugar in one twelve-ounce can of Pepsi).

INTERMEDIATE. Stop adding sugar to your food and limit yourself to three desserts a week. Gradually make those desserts less and less sweet.

ADVANCED. No more refined sugar, period! In any form. Raw honey, barley malt, maple syrup, maple sugar, rice syrup, and fruit juice—sweetened products are acceptable, but try not to overdo those.

MAKEOVER MANIAC. Eliminate everything sweet in your life, including reruns of *Full House*.

4. MEAT

BEGINNER. Allow yourself one portion of red meat or pork a day. This includes anything from a cow, pig, or lamb. (Don't be fooled by those "other white meat" ads for pork. Pork is nearly as dense as beef.) Also, don't become Mr. Venison, either. Add more fish and chicken to your diet.

INTERMEDIATE. Limit your red meat and pork consumption to three times a week. Try to eat only free-range poultry and meat whenever possible.

ADVANCED. Eliminate all red meat and pork from your diet. Make sure your poultry is free-range and your fish is from unpolluted waters whenever possible. Experiment with vegetarian meals.

MAKEOVER MANIAC. Eliminate meat completely from your life. Even counting sheep is forbidden.

5. DAIRY

BEGINNER. Become aware of how much dairy is in everything. Make one meal a day completely dairy-free.

INTERMEDIATE. Same as beginner, but pick one dairy product you eat often (milk, butter, cheese, yogurt, ice cream) and give it up completely. Try a dairy substitute instead.

ADVANCED. Give up all dairy products. Use dairy substitutes, but don't overdo it, as it may take a while for your body to clean out all the dairy.

MAKEOVER MANIAC. Spread the word. Try mooooning a Dairy Queen.

6. FOOD COMBINING

BEGINNER. Properly food combine one meal, preferably dinner, since you have more time in your day to digest an improperly combined breakfast or lunch. (See page 105.) And most importantly, pay attention to how your body responds to that meal compared to other meals.

INTERMEDIATE. Same as beginner, but make it two meals a day.

ADVANCED. Properly food combine all three meals, making lunch your protein meal most often.

MAKEOVER MANIAC. Properly combine your foods by color as well. For example, dark green vegetables with light spring-toned yellow carbohydrates. Avoid anything fuchsia. Also, make sure you eat everything in alphabetical order.

7. FAT

BEGINNER. Keep track of all the fat you are consuming. Count the number of fat grams you consume daily. Read the labels on processed food. Remember that the amount on the label is listed "per serving," so multiply that by "servings per container" if you eat the entire thing.

INTERMEDIATE. Cut your calculated fat intake by one-third. Try to use unsaturated fats from cold-pressed vegetable oils (especially olive, safflower, and canola) whenever possible.

ADVANCED. Only allow yourself fat from whole foods (fish, nuts, seeds, chicken, legumes, olives, avocados, etc.). Add to your food only cold-pressed vegetable oils and some margarines.

MAKEOVER MANIAC. Become so fat-free that SnackWell's wants to package you.

8. EXERCISE AND STRESS

BEGINNER. Walk one mile, at a comfortable pace, three times a week. Walk anywhere—the zoo, the park, the museum—but *not* the food court.

INTERMEDIATE. Walk and/or jog two miles, four days a week. Or do twenty to thirty minutes of any aerobic activity.

ADVANCED. Break a sweat every day with any aerobic activity, for at least twenty minutes. Add strength training two or three times a week, if possible.

MAKEOVER MANIAC. Dedicate your life to exercise! Each day of the week should be devoted to a different body part. If it's Tuesday, it must be deltoids. Also, spend one hour each day working on your Austrian accent.

9. SLEEP

BEGINNER. Become aware of your body's sleep patterns. Notice when your body needs sleep and also the times you sleep when you don't really need it, and *why*.

INTERMEDIATE. Same as beginner, plus try to establish healthy sleeping habits.

ADVANCED. Same as intermediate, plus keep a sleep journal to better track your pattern.

MAKEOVER MANIAC. Become so obsessed with your journal that you no longer have time to sleep.

10. GUSTO

BEGINNER. Read Chapter 13, "Gusto," once a week.

INTERMEDIATE. Same as beginner, plus find the gusto in one activity every day.

ADVANCED. Try to be in present time with everything you do. Enjoying the moment will help you have gusto throughout your day.

MAKEOVER MANIAC. Join every 12-step program you can. You must become one with Stuart Smalley!

For most of you, my ideas may seem a bit extreme (okay, maybe a lot extreme), but only at first glance. Everyone who initially asks me how to get started says, "I could never live without that," or "I'm not as disciplined as you are." In fact, I have had friends literally psych themselves right out of a successful attempt before they even get started. Eventually, they give in because they want to feel better, healthier, and more alive. I can't tell you how many people have said, "I wish I had listened to you twelve years ago!" So why should *you* act as your own roadblock to becoming healthier? There are plenty of other obstacles you'll need to navigate your way around, so at least cut yourself some slack by not being one of them from the start.

What Is Freedom?

Freedom, conceptually, is our God-given right. As American citizens, we are free to vote, free to choose religion; we have freedom of speech, and the list goes on and on. If you look up the word "free" in the dictionary, you will find that the meaning is "to emancipate, liberate, and gain independence." But you might be wondering to yourself, "What does this have to do with being healthier?" Okay, I'll tell you. Most of us weren't given many choices as young children. We were told what to eat, what we could wear to school, or even when to take a bath. When we were children, all those decisions were made for us. As we grew older, what was taught to us as a ritual became habitual, and most of us lived our lives pretty much the same way until we left home for the first time. For many of us, that's when we went off to college. This, of course, was the first time most of us could finally live an independent life. We were free to make our own choices and to live by those choices. Autonomy at last. What influenced our decisions the most was probably the behavior we learned as children. Either you went off on some opposite path out of spite, or you pretty much continued to live as you normally had. Your lack of discipline probably caused your greatest disappointments when you first left home. It's not anyone else's fault but your own. You made the choice, of your free will, to live whichever way you chose, or did you? Remember, *freedom* means to have liberated oneself from familiarity. We are creatures of habit, so were you free when you made those choices, or did you make them because you were most familiar and comfortable with the outcome? If it was the latter, than I would argue that you were not free at all but rather a prisoner of your habits. Freedom is having the knowledge of all your options and then making decisions based on what is best for your needs. A member of a cult has no freedom. She lives her life according to the ways of her group. How are you different from a cult member if you're still living the same way you did as a child?

This book is a journey to freedom. It will totally emancipate you from the horrible eating habits you never knew were bad for you. It will free you from the way you have been living your life because you "didn't know any better." That old excuse won't hold up anymore, because I am *finally* offering you a choice to make the decision to live a healthier new life . . . by exercising your own *free* will.

A Workable Program

This book is the culmination of a lot of experimenting over the years, and it offers a program I developed because each part of it is working for me. Over the past several years I have found that every person who tries *any* of the steps of my program sees positive results. I've encouraged friends like Michael Caine and Fran Drescher to try parts of this very program. When I was working with Michael Caine in *Noises Off* in 1991, he noticed that at lunchtime, I was eating as much if not more than anyone else, yet I was eating only certain foods. (I wasn't eating dairy and I was properly food combining.) He said to me, "How come you look so much better than you did on *Taxi* [which had ended eight years earlier] and you eat just as much as the rest of us but you have more energy than all of us put together? You're the only one not tired after lunch!" I told him that I had figured out a way of eating that helps me look like the "animal I was meant to be." He loved that concept so much that he wanted to know everything I did to get there. He was determined to become *his* best animal. He lost eighteen pounds in the eight weeks we worked together, and his skin and eyes absolutely glowed. (In fact, his beautiful wife, Shakira, came up to me at the wrap party and thanked me for turning her husband into an "animal.")

If you follow any part of this program you will definitely see results. Your energy level will come up and your weight will go down. Your skin will become healthier, and your life will be more balanced. There is no magic bullet here, and you may experience differences in your results, but I am certain that if you follow any or all of these ten steps, you'll like what you see in terms of progress, growth, and self-improvement. I've never seen it fail. I've never seen anyone who didn't feel better as a result of following any of these steps.

Take the time to read about each step and make your decision about what works for you. It doesn't really matter which step you decide to take first, and, *definitely*, the steps are not meant to be taken all at once! Experiment with each of the steps. It does not have to be all or nothing. I experimented for eight years! I've done the bulk of the trial-and-error work, so you won't have to guess too hard at your results. As the Nike ad says, *"Just do it!"*

When I started on this journey, I first gave up foods with chemicals, particularly the diet soda Tab. (Most people think I gave up dairy first because I'm so vocal about my crusade against all dairy products, but as you will soon find out, I'm pretty vocal about almost everything I'm passionate about.) I was drinking two of those big bottles (about a gallon) a day at the time, and I decided to give up all diet soda for two weeks. I figured that if I could do that, I would see how I felt and then decide whether I could "do this" the rest of my life. Sure enough, two weeks later, I drank my first Tab, and I felt all belchy and bloated. I could feel a real difference. I decided I was on the right path. I started reading every label, and pretty soon, chemical foods were out of my life. After a successful trial with giving up chemicals, I knew there had to be other foods I was eating that were affecting me adversely. So I continued on by giving up sugar, and then meat, and then dairy. I was constantly testing each step to see the effects and my body's response. Happily, the results always proved in my favor. Giving things up became easier for me as my body continued to respond so positively. My cravings for artificial substances dimmed and my body no longer needed the junk to feel good. In fact, the taste of chemicals became unappetizing. All this experimenting also opened my eyes to my freedom of choice instead of the confinement of my old habits, and once you try this program for yourself, I am certain you will experience the same exhilarating results.

Excuses, Excuses, Excuses!

What are *your* excuses for not being healthy?

- ❋ "I'm not sure where to start."
- ❋ "I'm a busy mom, and that's a full-time job."
- ❋ "I can't have it all."
- ❋ "I'm so tired all the time."
- ❋ "I just don't have the energy."
- ❋ "I just don't seem to have the time to work out."
- ❋ "I try to diet, but nothing seems to work."
- ❋ "My skin has always been bad."
- ❋ "Those dark circles under my eyes are because I have deep sockets."
- ❋ "I don't know what to eat."

The list could go on and on, I'm sure, but if you recognize any of those excuses, I'm here to tell you that you don't have to feel the way you do anymore. There is hope, and I'm here to help.

There will be many things in this book that you may never have heard before, or maybe they will be just a different explanation for things you thought you knew. Whether you decide to change any of the ten things that I changed in my life is completely up to you. You'll be better informed and a lot more aware of the areas in your life that might need help. I developed the following list of questions to help you identify those areas in your life that may need some adjustment. All these questions are addressed within these pages.

Marilu's Questions to Think About

Health

1. When was the last time you felt healthy?
2. Is there one area of your body that never feels healthy?
3. How often do you feel tired during the day?
4. How much do you sleep each night?
5. How do you identify stress in your body?
6. What do you do to get rid of stress?
7. Do you exercise regularly?
8. What is your definition of "balance" as it pertains to your life?
9. Where do you get your nutritional information?
10. Do you ask your doctor questions about your general health?
11. Do you understand your body's digestive system?
12. How often do you go to the bathroom every day?
13. What excuses do you give yourself for not living a healthy lifestyle?

Food

1. What is the difference between starch, protein, fat?
2. If you do not eat meat, do you know where you can get your protein?

3. Do you read the labels on the things you consume? Do you understand them?
4. What foods do you eat for flavor?
5. What foods do you eat for convenience?
6. What foods do you eat for weight loss?
7. What foods do you eat for health?
8. What foods do you eat for fun?
9. How do you feel physically after eating, salt, sugar, caffeine, alcohol, meat, dairy products?
10. How do these products make you feel mentally?
11. What is "good fat"?
12. What is "good cholesterol"?
13. What is an antioxidant?
14. What are nitrates? Nitrites? Sulfates?
15. What is Nutra Sweet? Equal? Sweet 'n Low?
16. What food do you eat more than any other?
17. What percentage of the food that you eat is not good for your health?
18. Do you skip breakfast? Why?
19. What foods do you snack on?
20. What percentage of your meals do you prepare at home?
21. What food items are always on your shopping list?
22. How often do you dine out?
23. In restaurants, what do you order most often?

Dieting

1. How often do you think about your weight?
2. How many times have you tried to lose weight by dieting?
3. Were you successful? Why or why not?
4. What were the circumstances that led you to take up a diet?
5. Have you ever been on a "desperation" diet? Why?
6. How often do you think about food during the day?
7. Do you eat certain foods "in secret"? What are they and why?
8. Do you binge on food? What moods lead you to this?

9. Do you use food to make yourself feel better? When?
10. Does your eating make you feel inadequate? How?
11. Are you ready and willing to control your eating?

Body Image

1. How often do you think about your body?
2. How does your body image affect your self-esteem?
3. Whom do you compare yourself to physically?
4. Do you long to have the same body you did at another time in your life? In what way?
5. What do you feel when you look in the mirror?
6. What is your best and worst feature?
7. What do you want to change about your appearance? Why? How would you like to do it?
8. How much time do you spend each day on your appearance?
9. What do you do everyday that makes you feel good about yourself?
10. What do you do everyday that makes you feel not so good about yourself?
11. Are you ready for your "TOTAL HEALTH MAKEOVER?"

What Is B.E.S.T.?

The word "best" conjures up different ideas for different people; it is a really subjective term. When I say "best," I think of an acronym: balance, energy, stamina, and toxin-free. When I was first asked to describe my program in a few words, I kept coming up with these concepts. To me, this whole book is about living a life filled with balance, energy, and stamina, which is also toxin-free. I kept repeating those words to my publisher, my friends, my family, and anyone else who would listen, and even a few who didn't! Then one day it hit me. Those four words spell out "best."

The positive message of showing people how to be their own best was enough motivation for me to put these thoughts down on paper. I really live my life this way. I walk my talk, and continue to strive every day to be my best, and I'd like you to be your best, too. I want you to feel as good as I do, and no matter who you are, it's not impossible, nor is it too late for you to start. If you remember only one thing from this book, please remember always to strive to be the B.E.S.T. you can be. You are a work in progress. Never give up.

"Somewhere over the Rainbow..." — My Rainbow Theory

I could change the words to that famous song so easily. Anyone who knows me has without a doubt heard my "Rainbow Theory" at least once. I give new meaning to the phrase "chasing rainbows"! I came up with this theory a few years back, and even told it on *Late Night with David Letterman*. It's a perfect description of what most of us go through in the cycles of our lives.

I used to go on long walks and runs with my brother Tommy when I lived in Los Angeles during the early 1980s. We would have great talks, and one day I realized that there had to be a way to describe the cycle I was continually finding myself going through in my quest to lose weight and get fit. One day, I launched into this idea that all the colors in a rainbow correlated perfectly to that vicious cycle.

Try to picture in your mind a rainbow, each color illuminated vivid and bright. In my theory, each of the colors represents a different period and behavioral pattern in your life. You wake up one morning and you say to yourself, "That's it! Today I am starting my new fitness program, and this time, *nothing* can stop me!" You are in the Purple phase. Come hell or high water, you're going to stick to the program with pure perfection. You make a vow to work out every day, eat perfectly, not drink any alcohol, get the right amount of sleep. You're even going to floss . . . twice! It's cattle-prod-to-the-brain time. You become an anal-retentive, obsessive maniac. And then one day you wake up and realize you're starting to feel really good about your progress, and it might be okay to become a little social again. You're moving into the Blue phase.

As humans, we are inherently social animals, and besides, you feel so good about your success in Purple, you want to show it off a little bit in Blue, you know what I mean? So you start going out a little more, and you're a little bit nervous because you don't want to fall off your program. You are a deliberately cautious Blue: You go out, but you don't completely enjoy yourself because you're worried that you might not get up and work out the next day. Then one day you wake up and you're feeling perfectly balanced. Everything in your life is in its place, and you have entered the often-strived-for phase of Green.

People who are in Green can hang out with anyone at any stage of the rainbow. They are the epitome of the perfect blend of discipline and chaos. Everything is organic in their lives. They can socialize without tipping the scale and feel really good about themselves. Unfortunately, this phase doesn't last very long. You wake up one day and realize that your Green has turned to Yellow, which really means that your "balance" is getting unbalanced and is tilting toward the other end of the rainbow.

A Yellow can fake being a Green, but not for long. A little more black starts creeping into your wardrobe to hide the slight weight gain. (Of course, New Yorkers always wear black, so this is not a true indicator in some parts of the country.) As a Yellow, you're starting to do more *talking* about your workouts than actually working out. You're booking social dinners *and* lunches, leaving very little room in your life for any type of healthy discipline. You're simply sliding into the world of Orange.

Orange is when your social life has consumed any and all focus you had on your physical well-being. You know you haven't been to the gym in weeks, and you're so bloated from eating and drinking, even your black jeans make you look fat! And flossing? You're lucky you brush! You're a total party animal now; lunches, dinners, and happy hour buffets. Before you know it, you're in Red, and in Red, you're either lying on the floor with drool coming out of your mouth . . . or you're in Italy.

> *The way I see it, if you want the rainbow, you gotta put up with the rain.*
>
> DOLLY PARTON

You'll know when you've had your fill of Red, because one day you'll wake up, look in the mirror, and say to yourself, "back to Purple." The pendulum will swing all the way around the color spectrum. People never seem to back up a color. They get to the end and swing around to the beginning.

I know you recognize your own behavior within this theory, but probably never thought of it this way. Think of all the fun you'll have at your next party trying to explain my Rainbow Theory to your friends. Hey, it's good for a laugh, and you'll probably agree with its validity. I have been at Green lately, writing this book and doing *Chicago*, but I still go through the rainbow, and you know, there's one thing I tell you for sure. There is no pot of gold at the end of that rainbow, only a pot belly and a sign that reads: "This Way to Purple! → → "

2 | Balance

*H*ave you ever noticed that whenever you eat something very salty, you crave something very sweet afterward? It's no accident that this invariably happens. It's your body's way of trying to balance the food you eat. My entire program is predicated on the concept that your body is always seeking balance. The relationship you have with food and your ability to understand its effects on your body will greatly impact how well you are balanced both in your diet and as a person. Throughout this book, I will describe this constant theme of balance because, to me, not only is that the real purpose of this book (helping you to live a more balanced life), but it is the way I seek to live my own life.

My entire program is based on the law of nature that everything in the universe vacillates between two major forces, expansive and contractive energy. These two forces are complementary opposites, and everything exists in a constant state of flux between these two forces. For every action, there is an opposite and equal reaction. This is a law of nature. It cannot be changed. You may have heard the terms "yin" and "yang" to describe these opposite forces, but you can use any number of word combinations to describe the same principle: up/down, cold/hot, light/dark, female/male, push/pull, passive/active. All these combinations describe the same phenomenon known as yin (expansive) and yang (contractive). Everything in the universe exists between these two forces of nature. There is nothing that is set in a fixed state. Everything is constantly moving.

TYPICAL YIN-YANG QUALITIES APPLIED TO HUMAN PERSONALITY AND PHYSIOLOGY

YANG	YIN
Outgoing	Introverted
Active	Passive
Masculine	Feminine
Positive	Negative
Focused mind	Serene
Hyperactive mentality	Unclear, dreamy
Aggressive	Timid
Angry, impatient	Fearful, insecure
Loud voice	Soft voice
Urgent	Tardy
Logical	Intuitive
Quick	Slow
Desire-filled	Complacent
Tense, strong body	Flaccid, weak body
Red complexion	Pale complexion
Warmer body and personality	Cooler body and personality
Dry skin and less body fluid	Moist skin and more body fluid

Because life has so many fluctuations, it's better for us not to live in the extremes, but rather more toward the center of those extremes. Life is crazy enough as it is, so if we try to live in the extremes, we live in an erratic state. The feast-or-famine, all-or-nothing syndrome creates more chaos than order. Nature will always strive for a balance. It is as if there were an imaginary pendulum swinging between the opposing forces of nature.

Imagine living your life in Room A, which is consistently between 68 and 72 degrees, compared to living in Room B, which constantly fluctuates between 100 degrees and 32 degrees. In Room B, just when you can no longer stand the heat, you are grateful for the sudden drop in temperature to 32 degrees. You actually crave freezing temperatures—until *that* becomes unbearable, and you then crave abnormally high temperatures. In both rooms, a balance is reached, but Room B puts the body through unnecessary stress and exhaustion.

How we do everything in our lives can be compared to this. All things try to become balanced. For the most part, we choose how we go about finding that balance: thrashing back and forth between extremes, or mildly rocking back and forth close to life's fulcrum. One keeps us stressed and tired, the other keeps us energized and nearly stress-free. Not all things in life are our choice, though. We can't always do everything near the center. We are forced to deal with extremes that are beyond our control—job deadlines, being fired, divorce, a death in the family. If we have filled our lives with the more centered behavior that we *do* have control over, we will be much better prepared (more energetic, level-headed, etc.) to handle the extreme elements in life that we *don't* have control over. It's up to you to decide how far you want your lifestyle pendulum to swing. Do you want to live your life in extremes (a drug addict or a hermit), or aim for a more balanced (not necessarily boring) life? Living in extremes takes its toll. The show business world I live in can be very extreme at times, but trying to remain centered as a person helps me cope with all the ups and downs and twists and turns.

We all know people who are so set in their ways that they are unyielding to the slightest change that might rock their world. Then, of course, there are those people who float through life with their heads in the clouds, completely unaware that life is going on around them. Think about the people you know who fit these descriptions. How would they handle a good or bad event like winning the lottery or losing a family member? How well do you think they would be able to cope? These extreme types of people probably won't do very well at dealing with extreme circumstances.

Understanding Extreme Foods

When I first started studying about food, I discovered that all food could be placed on a number line that classifies food from yin (expansive) to yang (contractive). All food can be divided into three categories, each having its appropriate place on that number line. Animal foods, such as meat, fish, dairy, and eggs, are very yang and therefore fall under the contractive end of the line. (You'll notice that after you eat these foods, you often feel contracted. They have that effect on your body!) Plant derivatives, like sugar, spices, alcohol, and even drugs, are very yin, and therefore fall on the expansive end. (You'll feel expanded, bloated, and puffy after you eat these foods.) The third group is plant foods, like fruits and vegetables and grains, which lie in the middle between the two extremes. A balanced diet will focus primarily on eating these types of foods. There are also varying degrees of each extreme. For example, red meat is a really concentrated food, and that makes it more contractive than chicken, which is still contrac-

3. PLANT DERIVATIVES | **2. PLANT FOODS** | **1. ANIMAL FOODS**

drugs · alcohol · sugar | fruits · vegetables · grains · seeds | cheese · eggs · fish · chicken · meat

EXPANSIVE — **CONTRACTIVE**

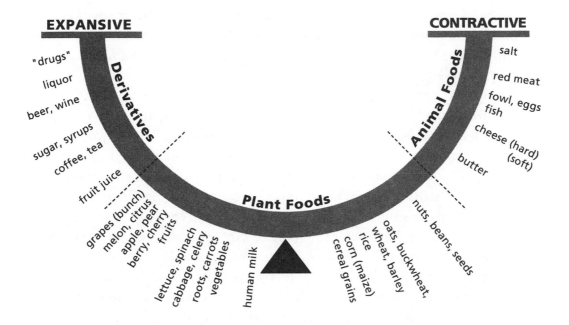

EXPANSIVE

"drugs"

liquor

beer, wine

sugar, syrups

coffee, tea

fruit juice

Derivatives

grapes (bunch)
melon, citrus
apple, pear
berry, cherry
fruits

lettuce, spinach
cabbage, celery
roots, carrots
vegetables

human milk

Plant Foods

oats, buckwheat,
wheat, barley
rice
corn (maize)
cereal grains

nuts, beans, seeds

Animal Foods

butter

cheese (hard)
(soft)

fish

fowl, eggs

red meat

salt

CONTRACTIVE

tive, but not as concentrated. Likewise, cheese is more concentrated than milk, so it, too, is more contractive. (It takes up to ten pounds of milk to make one pound of cheese!) Plant derivatives are usually made from the most expansive part of the plant, so it makes sense that they would have an expansive reaction on our behavior. The more processed the food is, the more expansive it is. Drugs are the most extreme expansive element you can put into your body, and the more extreme the drug, the more expansive it is. Plant foods can also have extremes, but they don't tax your body or your digestion as much as the other two groups. Nuts, beans, and grains are more contractive than grapes, melons, and other fruits, which tend to be more expansive.

I definitely used to have extreme cravings. As soon as I satisfied one extreme, I automatically craved the other. When I was a child, I constantly went back and forth between a salty pretzel (yang) and a sugary Twizzler (yin). Before I started eating the way I do now, after a very heavy meat meal (yang), the first thing I wanted was a sugary, puffy, creamy, dessert (yin). Why do you think bars put out free salty peanuts? They know that the salty nuts (yang) will get you to drink alcohol (yin). As I've changed my diet, I still get cravings, but my choices were much closer to the center as I became a more balanced eater. As I moved toward the center of the number line, I noticed that I also felt better.

I realize that all this might seem a bit overwhelming (maybe even confusing?) at first, but once you get the hang of it, you'll easily be able to identify the food you eat according to these terms. "Expansive" and "contractive" are easy universal terms to understand. Everything about being healthy can be described according to the general principles of yin and yang as well. Relationships, work, performing, even parenting (giving your child the balance of freedom and parameters), you name it, it fits. But it is important to understand that the pendulum between yin and yang is in constant motion even if the swings are slight.

Balance in Your Diet

Maintaining a centered (or balanced) diet is the most natural approach to eating, but most people eat an extreme diet. Experts agree that eating meat and sugar in the amounts that most Americans do increases physical hypertension and high blood pressure, which also leads to an increase in heart disease. These ailments afflict one-third of the American adult population. People usually eat foods that they crave to satisfy both their hunger and their craving. Generally speaking, that pendulum is usually in full swing for most people. Our diets tend to be full of variety, and the tremendous amount of food that we have to choose from is staggering! While creating balance is important to strive for in all areas of your life, you can start by creating balance in your diet. Food is a part of everyone's life and it is an easy way to explain my concept on balance.

The first rule of thumb is to understand that opposites attract. Extremely expansive foods can only be balanced by eating something extremely contractive. (It works the other way around, too!) It's like being on a seesaw. What goes up must come down, and it's the same thing with your diet. On one end sit contractive foods, and on the other end are expansive foods. To balance that seesaw, you should try to eat the foods that reside in the middle. If you are eating an unbalanced

> *The average American will eat 240 pounds of meat, 126 pounds of sugar, and less than 10 pounds of whole grain per year.*

diet, then you are living an unbalanced lifestyle. Of course, the definition of what a "balanced" diet is has drastically changed since I was a kid. We were your typical meat-and-potatoes Midwestern family. (Talk about bad food combining and extreme foods!) Today, I am able to teach my two sons a whole new approach to eating a healthy and balanced meal, and I can also teach them at a very young age *how* they should approach food and eating. From the moment my kids sat in a high chair and had solid food for the first time, I wanted them to be able to touch it, taste it, smell it, *and* put it in their mouths. (As long as it was food that they couldn't choke on.) I wanted them to feed themselves so that they could learn their own rhythm. I didn't want to be one of those mothers

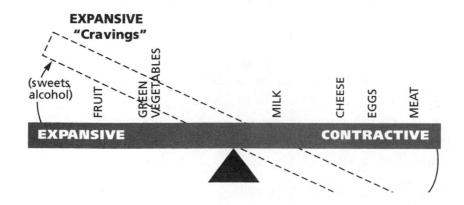

who just shoveled food into her children's mouths. I knew that would only lead to problems for that baby later in life. You have to let children discover their own rhythm of eating. And since infants can't choose the food they eat, as the parent, you can give them control over their intake. Amazingly, children will eat if they're hungry and won't if they're full. Instilling in them at a young age a good relationship with food is so important. But it's never too late to rediscover that relationship as an adult, either.

Food and Behavior

Have you ever noticed that you might get a little cranky if you go without eating too long? Likewise, have you ever eaten so much that you get sleepy? These are pretty common scenarios that illustrate that our behavior is absolutely influenced by the food we eat. Under this assumption, it makes a lot of sense that the more extreme the food is, the more extreme the behavior will be. Think about someone who has had too much sugar and goes buzzing around until that "high" wears off, and he becomes a lethargic slug. Eating an extreme diet makes it harder for us to control our behavior. We become increasingly tense, frustrated, and basically out of control. I remember reading a study a few years back about how a maximum-security prison greatly reduced the violence rate when the prisoners were not allowed to eat meat (a very contractive and extreme food) or sugar (a very expansive and extreme food). There is a lot of evidence that food triggers a behavioral response in people. Eating an extreme diet not only affects a person's behavior but also limits their performance in every aspect of their lives. If your body is in a state of imbalance, it will try to compensate in some way to swing that pendulum back around to the center. If you eat an extreme yin diet (expansive), you will find yourself in a state of overexpansion. Your behavior will be too open and detached from reality. These are the people who seem to just float through life with no direction. They're victims of their own behavior.

People who eat a very yang diet (contractive) are just the opposite. They are very closed off, and are often tense and uptight. These people are absolute control freaks, and are always trying to maintain some sense of order and control over their (as well as others') lives. They're rigid in their thinking and approach to everything they do.

So what should you eat? Maintaining a healthy centered diet primarily consisting of whole, natural, good-quality (preferably organic) food will help keep you in top form. Be aware of what you're eating. So many people eat without even thinking about it! (Personally, I love to love my food!) When you don't pay attention to what you're eating, you aren't paying attention to the effects of what you're eating. A big part of creating balance in your life is being aware of the extremes and familiar with where your center resides.

Eating an extreme diet can have another side effect that is equally unpleasant although hardly life-threatening (except to your loved ones). It's known to cause personal hygiene problems such as offensive body odor and extremely smelly stool. This is especially true of people who eat a lot of meat, dairy, and sugar in their diets. Eating a more centered diet and better-quality food will help minimize the malodorous effects.

Changing Your Palate

One of the things that I discovered early on in my newfound adventure of recreating myself and my health was that I never really took the time to taste my food. I would put too much salt on my meat or sugar on my cereal, because those flavors were the only things my palate could taste. As I worked toward centering my diet and simplifying my food choices, I went on a kick of not only trying to taste the food I was eating, but also trying to dissect each and every aspect of it. If I ate an apple, I wanted to savor the taste of the meat, the skin, the core, and the juice individually. Together, these were the elements that made an apple taste like an apple. I wanted to know the difference in the flavors of each element. This experiment proved helpful in teaching me the principle of changing my palate, or reprogramming my taste buds.

Think of an artist's palette, which prominently displays the many colors the artist will use in creating his work of art. Each color represents a piece of the final masterpiece. On the palette, they are merely colors. Together on the artist's canvas, they become art. Do you really taste your food? When was the last time you actually tasted the simple grain flavors in a piece of bread? (Or do you need butter and jelly to give the bread any flavor?) Our tongues (or palate) have become so assaulted by the strong tastes of salt and sugar that they can't taste anything else. They have become anesthetized in a way to the more wonderful subtle flavors of the simpler foods that are not salted or sugared.

Taste in food is very important. We all love food that tastes good, but our taste buds have become so desensitized that we can only taste extreme flavors. Certain extreme foods such as fats, meats, sweets, and processed foods will satisfy the immediate desire for certain tastes, but after a while, your taste buds become immune to tasting flavors. For you to taste anything, the flavors have to become stronger and stronger. I have a friend who has to add a lot of salt and chili pepper to everything, otherwise he literally can't taste a thing. In addition, sweets must be overly sugary for him to taste anything sweet. An ordinary oatmeal cookie has absolutely no flavor to him. Are you the kind of person who automatically reaches for the salt shaker before you even taste your food? Or adds spoonfuls of sugar to presweetened cereal?

How you taste food is important to creating balance in your diet. The first step to changing your palate is recognizing whether your palate has been numbed and your tongue swollen from years of extreme flavors and extreme foods. To change your palate, you have to eliminate the culprits causing the problems. Get rid of your salt shaker at the table. Things will start to taste different to you because you will start to taste flavors other than "salt." If you have a sweet tooth, try cutting back on the sugary flavors that have been destroying your palate for years. Try less sugar in your coffee and in your cereal, and if you must eat desserts, try picking ones that are less and less sweet (such as choosing a plain donut instead of a glazed one, or skipping the icing on the cake). As you eliminate extreme foods and extreme flavors from your diet, you will eventually be able to rediscover foods that you haven't "tasted" in years.

The Art of Chewing

The way you eat is an expression of who you are. (I always say you can tell *a lot* about a man by the way he eats.) Eating begins with the simple task of chewing. You might think that you've got this one down, but many people don't. Would you rather have a shovel than a fork when eating? Do you play "beat the clock" when you sit down for a meal? Do you eat so quickly that you don't realize you're full until you're stuffed? Do you notice visible remnants of last night's dinner in your morning stool? If you said "yes" to any one of these questions, then I've got news for you:

YOU HAVE TO LEARN TO CHEW YOUR FOOD!

The best visual I can give you to help remind you of the importance of thoroughly chewing your food is that *your stomach does not have teeth!* Digestion starts the second you begin to chew. You will completely mess up your digestive system by not chewing your food efficiently. Chewing your food properly will also help you to taste and disseminate all the luscious and delicious flavors in each and every morsel of food you put into your mouth. I have a saying: "Drink your food and chew what you drink." That does not mean, however, drink a liquid with your food. It means that your food should be liquid before you swallow it and your drinks should be tasted before you swallow them. Chewing is a multifunctional process. Mechanically, it helps break up the food we eat and enables chemicals in our saliva to begin the digestion process. Chewing also stimulates the flow of gastric juices. Whole vegetable foods and whole grains *must* be chewed until liquefied to release their full nutritional value. If you don't chew your food properly, you will inevitably feel lethargic, gassy, and undernourished. This is why so many people, even though they are eating large amounts of food all day, are still hungry. Their bodies are not properly receiving the nutrients from the food that has been eaten because the food has not been chewed to a form that the stomach can recognize and break down. Your stomach cannot "work" on whole pieces of food. Therefore, the pieces pass through your system undigested. You should chew each bite of food thirty to fifty times to know that you have effectively chewed your food. However, that seems difficult, especially at first. So aim for twenty to twenty-five chews per bite instead of the typical four to six. Believe me, you will eventually lose your self-consciousness about this as you become an expert discreet chewer. Chewing your food well also helps slow you down in the eating process. Dining can become a stress-free and enjoyable experience instead of a wolf-it-down-as-fast-as-you-can, bloaty, belchy encounter.

❋ ❋ ❋ ❋ ❋ ❋ ❋ ❋ ❋ ❋

MARILU'S FIVE TIPS ON HOW TO EAT

- **Dine when you eat. Take the time to enjoy your meal.**
- **Increase your eating awareness. Taste what you're eating!**
- **Chew your food well.**

- Don't drink anything with your meal. If you must drink, make sure you sip. Have something to drink fifteen to twenty minutes before or an hour after eating.

- Eat only when you're hungry.

❋   ❋   ❋   ❋   ❋   ❋   ❋   ❋   ❋   ❋

Food for Thought

To realize a truly "centered" or "balanced" diet, I thought it was a good idea to take things back to a basic understanding of what food really is. Proteins, carbohydrates, and fats are not foods, but rather nutritional categories into which all foods fall. All three are essential to a well-balanced lifestyle, and are the primary sources of fuel for our body. They can be difficult to understand, so here's a quick review of what each of these categories is and the types of foods that fit each of them.

Protein

Protein literally means "primary substance," which is a perfect definition since all tissues in our bodies are built and repaired with protein. The main function of protein is the formation of body protein and new cells. The antibodies of the immune system, most hormones, the hemoglobin of red blood cells, and all enzymes have protein as their basic component. It is the major source of building the necessary materials for muscles, blood, skin, hair, nails, and our internal organs, like the brain and the heart. Next to water, protein is more plentiful than any other substance in the body. Protein can be used as a source of heat and energy for the body at a rate of four calories per gram.

Some hormones in the body are proteins, such as the thyroid hormone and insulin. These control several bodily functions, such as growth, sexual development, and metabolism.

Carbohydrates

Carbohydrates are the best source of energy for all bodily functions, especially the brain and central nervous system. They also help with muscle exertion and assist in the digestion and assimilation of foods. Carbohydrates come from plant sources and, like protein, each gram is four calories. A carbohydrate is made up of the chemical elements carbon, hydrogen, and oxygen. These chemicals provide us with immediately available calories by producing heat in the body when the carbon unites with the oxygen in your bloodstream. They also help regulate protein and fat metabolism because fat requires carbohydrates to break down within the liver. This is very important for dieters to remember when they mistakenly think they should eliminate carbohydrates from their diet. Fat can only "burn" in a carbohydrate "flame."

All sugars and starches are carbohydrates. Complex carbohydrates (starchy foods) take longer to break down enzymes in the body. You may have heard the term "empty calories" already; it refers to carbohydrates that lack essential vitamins, minerals, and fibers. White-flour cookies, candy, cakes, and other starchy sweet foods all fall into this category. A diet that is too extreme in these foods will probably result in a nutritional deficiency as well as a weight problem. Although you might get a quick boost of energy from eating snacks that are these types of carbohydrates (they cause a sudden rise in blood-sugar levels), you might feel the effects when that "buzz" wears off, like dizziness, fatigue, nervousness, or a headache.

Carbohydrates can be manufactured in the body from some amino acids. Most authorities agree that 55–60 percent of total calories should be from complex carbohydrates, with a minimum of 100 grams a day being essential. This is so different from the old diet I went on as a teenager, where the recommendation was 25 grams a day! (No wonder I was carbohydrate starved!) Of course, individual differences in metabolism, the amount of exercise you do, and your weight will have a bearing on what your individual needs are.

Fat

Fats—or lipids—are the most concentrated source of energy in our diets. There are three classes of fats: triglycerides, phospholipids, and sterols. When oxidized, fats furnish more than twice the number of calories per gram as carbohydrates or proteins. One gram of fat yields nine calories to the body. The function of fat is vital, but too much can be a major health problem, so finding that proper balance is essential to a "centered" diet. Standard American dietary guidelines suggest that the total fat intake should not exceed 30 percent of the day's total food intake. I strongly believe that it should be much lower, between 20 percent and 25 percent. I have very strong opinions on fat and its place in the diet. I have devoted an entire chapter in this book (Chapter 10) to a more in-depth look at fat. Meanwhile, the charts on the next page will help you identify the differences between carbohydrates, fats, protein, and alkaline-forming foods.

Balancing/Centering Your Body

As a dancer, one of the most important things I strive for is "finding my center." Everything a dancer does is concentrated in the center of her body, which stems from the stomach area. When I talk about balance, I'm not just talking about food or diet. The way you carry your body (your posture) speaks volumes about the balance you have in your life. If you were to look at yourself from a side view, imagine seeing a line that runs down the center of your body. What is in front of that line should be equal to what is behind that line. The bigger the front, the bigger the back. That is why you rarely see someone with rounded shoulders who doesn't have a pot belly. Your posture is an indication of your personality, and like your diet, it correlates with what's going on with your body. If your posture is centered and balanced, you are more likely to be a centered and balanced person. On the other hand, if your posture is slouchy and distorted, something is out of balance.

EXAMPLES OF B.E.S.T. NUTRITIONAL FOODS

CARBOHYDRATES

Whole grains

Maple sugar and syrup
   raw honey

Fruits

Vegetables

FAT

Margarine

Vegetable oils

Whole grains

PROTEIN

Fish and poultry

Soybean products

Eggs

Whole grains

WATER

Fruits

Vegetables

Beverages

ACID-FORMING FOODS

Legumes

Beans

Chickpeas

Lentils

Catsup

Mustard

Olives

Coffee

Cocoa

Alcohol

Milk

Meat

Oatmeal

Pasta

Eggs

Fish

Plums

Prunes

Cranberries

Cornstarch

Flour products

Noodles

Organ meats

Asparagus

Brussels sprouts

**ALKALINE-FORMING
FOODS**

Vegetables

Fruits

Molasses

Maple syrup

Honey

Dates, raisins

Soy, figs

Grapes

Grapefruits

Lemons

Melons

Corn

Millet

Our bodies are made up of zillions of cells, and in the simplest of terms, each cell's function is to have something go in, something get processed, and something come out. When we are out of balance, this process can be interrupted and the processing part of the equation gets stuck, so nothing comes out. The cells become traumatized and tend to hoard, thereby interrupting the elimination process. A good example of this hoarding occurred when I would stay up all night to write a term paper in high school. I'd jump on the scale the next morning thinking I had lost weight from burning extra calories all night, when in fact I had gained two pounds even though I didn't eat anything! It was years later that I discovered that this happened because my body needed to balance the trauma of having to stay up all night. Sometimes our bodies hoard when we are dieting because they haven't balanced out the changes we've introduced. Don't worry, your body is a highly sophisticated machine that tries to make sense out of everything you do to it. Don't panic, sometimes it just takes a while.

The balancing act your body sometimes goes through can be compared to the sanitation system you set up for your home. If you have garbage cans and garbage bags and you've set up a procedure for removing the garbage from your home, your sanitation system will be working properly. If, however, you let garbage pile up, your living space will be overrun with clutter and unnecessary waste. You need to learn how to keep your sanitation system in good working order. Remember, something goes in, something gets processed, and something comes out: This is simply balance brought down to the molecular level. Everything in life is about balance and the centering between the two opposing forces of yin and yang.

3 | Taking the Plunge

I have often said that I could never have written this book fifteen, ten, or even five years ago, because most people weren't aware enough of the connection between their lifestyles and their health. Fifteen years ago people didn't know a fat gram from a graham cracker. There was no such thing as food labeling, so exactly what was in that can of soup was the $64,000 question. And soy? That was often confused with a Yiddish exclamation. Thankfully, the world is more educated now, and I really believe that people are finally ready to make important changes in their eating habits, in their commitment to exercise, and in creating a more positive attitude about themselves. We are striving for a more balanced lifestyle these days, though it's important to remember one thing: You didn't get fat or unhealthy overnight, so you shouldn't expect to get thin and healthy overnight. But it won't take you long to feel a difference.

Making the Commitment

The secret to living a longer, healthier life can be learned. Choosing to "take that first step" is something only you can do for yourself. What I want to accomplish in this book is to tell you the ten steps I took to change my health, and to explain why I took each step. Once *you* know, you can't choose not to know anymore. You can choose to ignore it, but sooner or later, the reality of maintaining your unhealthy lifestyle will catch up with you. Anyone who is still eating an unnatural, artificial diet that consists of processed and synthesized foods is making a choice to be an inferior version of himself or herself. You would never consider using faulty or low-quality materials to make your home. Why would you *ever* choose faulty low-quality "materials" to make your body?

> *Insanity is doing the same thing over and over again, but expecting different results.*
>
> RITA MAE BROWN

Now that you've made a commitment to try some new ideas, I can't stress to you enough that this program takes time and experimentation to really achieve an overall total health makeover. It's a very gradual process that combines the mind, body, and spirit, so as you progress, some results won't be as tangible as others. You'll notice an improvement in the measurable aspects such as weight, skin, and even stamina relatively fast. Areas such as creating less stress in your life and adjusting your gusto might take a little longer to see on a day-to-day basis, but you'll notice the overall effect when you finally start to strike that balance. Although you will feel significant changes quickly by taking any one of these steps, it can take up to a year to convert your broken-down organs into new healthy ones.

As I've said before, these ten steps aren't meant to be taken all at once. It would be senseless for anyone to attempt such a task, not to mention completely unhealthy. It has taken me years to reach this balanced state of health, and a lot of trial and error. But once I made up my mind to start down this path, I knew I would never go back to my old ways.

Before I started this program, I *thought* I looked good (once in a while) and I *felt* really healthy (most of the time). But deep down, I knew I didn't feel right and that I was doing something wrong. I just didn't know how to get myself out of it. I felt trapped. At the time, I had nothing else to compare it to until I started to experiment with these ten steps. I think that people who make only small adjustments in their diet and lifestyle are in the worst situation. They haven't made enough of a change to feel the results, yet they have made a big enough change to feel deprived. I assure you that even if you think you're feeling really good right now, I can help you to feel better. How great would that be?

> A recent University of California, San Francisco study showed that for most people it is easier to make big changes in diet and lifestyle than it is to make moderate ones.

The first step in taking better care of *you* is identifying what is right in your life. As a teenager (and well into my adulthood) whenever I wanted to look at myself objectively, I would make a list of all the good and bad things in my life. The good list became known as the "Good Nails" list because the first thing on this list was always my good nails. (I gave up biting my nails for Lent when I was thirteen.) On the other hand, my bad list became known as the "TBM" list ("Things Bothering Me"), because I never saw the bad things as permanent, but rather as things I could change or improve. It doesn't matter what kind of list you make, but before you get started, go back and take a look at your answers to the questionnaire in Chapter 1. Honestly assess the areas in your life that you're pleased with, and those you would like to improve upon. Ask yourself how you *should* be living your life so that you have more of a balance. If you are in pain or have any discomfort in your daily routine, what can you change or improve? Are you under so much stress that at the end of the day you can't think straight? Are you getting enough exercise? Do you drink too much coffee? Do you think that hot dogs, pizza, and Big Macs are your *only* choices for lunch? You have to acknowledge that there is a problem before you can execute a proper solution. That's true for any area of your life. *Your health is the single most important factor in your life.* It's the basis from which every other aspect of your life stems. Without it, you're nothing. (Except sick or dead.) You can have all the money in the world, you can have all the power in the world, but disease doesn't discriminate. You have been dealt a certain hand in life, and you have been given all the opportunity to play that hand the best you can. Everything you need to live a longer, happier, healthier life is literally at your fingertips (including this book, for starters).

By now you know that a short-term solution never lasts because it doesn't teach you to be in control. It controls you. A quick-weight-loss diet is a perfect example. You aren't in control of how that program works, nor can you choose which foods to eat. All you know is that if you follow that program you should lose weight. But how long can you stay on that program, or keep off those pounds? And what exactly have you learned? Your old unhealthy habits creep right back into your life, and you are back to square one. Unhappy, unhealthy, and on another diet. A person who lives in constant deprivation and with constant resentment can never truly be healthy (or happy). That person is continually seeking a "quick fix" for her heartburn, her headache, and those extra ten-plus pounds. You name it, they've got a fast, albeit temporary, solution. Wouldn't it be great to live a life where you never had to think about a remedy because you rarely have an ailment? To never "diet" again because you are finally in control? You can, and now is the time to take that first step.

> *Learning is suddenly understanding something you've understood all your life, but in a new way.*
>
> DORIS LESSING

Detoxification and Healing Crises

Know what you're getting yourself into, and you'll know where you're going. As you embark on this adventure to health, you should know that you might encounter some bumps in the road along the way. (That's why it's an adventure. How boring would a smooth and paved road be, anyway?)

As you start to cleanse yourself of all your toxins, your body will need to readjust itself to its new healthier existence. This process is often referred to as the detoxification cycle. The name is far worse than the actual event. Don't get this vision of an alcoholic going through all the pain and suffering of getting clean and sober. You won't be hunched in a corner, shaking uncontrollably, with drool coming from your mouth. Your body will naturally go through a reversal process that undoes the damage you have created over many, many years. New tissue, which is healthy, strong, virile, and active, replaces old diseased and corrupted tissue. Each cell in your body is like a little unit of life. So if you've been polluting or destroying those cells in any way, you are depleting your "power supply."

You may not realize that cells divide themselves rather than "multiply." That division is not infinite, however. As you develop, certain cells take on specialized functions. They become allmighty protectors. Once your permanent cells are established, all your other cells become transient. Those on the surface are replaced much faster than those found more deeply within your body.

Part of the reason I'm giving you this information is so that you'll realize and appreciate the importance of keeping your body in good working order. Your body is a well-oiled machine that, when functioning properly, works as a whole unit. Even though you have individual organs all operating independently, if everything goes right, you're never aware of it. When something goes wrong, however, it seems to cause a chain reaction. The detoxification process works under the same principle. Correcting the areas of your body that are dysfunctional will cause a chain reaction until each area works as it should. Consider this detoxing as a cleansing of the body and a time for rebirth and rejuvenation. It is a period where your body rids itself of unwanted, unneeded, and unhealthy materials. Elimination is not accomplished just by going to the bathroom. To do this effectively, you have to replace all those polluted cells and infested molecules with healthy new ones. And to accomplish that task, you have to deliberately render those old cells inactive and rid your body of their harmful aftereffects. You need to create a new "how to live" program for yourself and replace those old "ineffective" habits in the process.

Detoxification mostly happens at night. It is basically a two-step "taking out the trash" process. The first step allows the "trash" living in your body to be easily picked up. The molecules become "sticky" or "activated," making them more dangerous than they were when they were dormant. Now that they've been activated you may experience an even worse withdrawal reaction. You don't want these molecules hanging around for too long. Step two gets rid of the unwanted "trash" in a timely manner. "Conjunction" occurs when the sticky molecules are picked up by tiny little carrier molecules and are rendered "inactive" as they are carried away. They become more soluble in the water of your blood or bile and leave your body through either your kidneys or your intestine.

Some of the toxins in your body that you'll be flushing through your detoxification are aluminum, lead, caffeine, nicotine, dairy, and preservatives found in food, just to name a few. With every toxin you attack, your body will have some physical reaction as it adjusts itself to its "toxin-free" environment. This is when you may have a "healing crisis," that is, you may experience many different types of side effects as a result of your healing. For example, a commonly known side effect of giving up caffeine is what is often referred to as a "caffeine headache," which lasts about four days or until your craving for caffeine subsides. When you give up dairy, you may notice a runny nose for a few days. Because our bodies have many different orifices, we get rid of toxins not only by going to the bathroom but by releasing them through the bronchial tubes, the skin, and the lymphatic system as well. You can't always anticipate the consequences of a well-intended effort to change long and hard-to-break habits. You can, however, realize that the side effects are a temporary condition that leads you to a more permanent and healthier way of life. Don't get scared by what I'm telling you here, because whether you are aware of it or not, you have gone through this process many times before. Every time you started a diet or changed your habits in any way, your body adjusted in some way, whether it was extra elimination, nervous energy, lightheadedness, fatigue, and so on—you just never knew what to call it before. I hope this time will be the last time you ever have to go through this. Please note that not everyone will experience a healing crisis. It won't happen to you unless you're out of balance to begin with. The intensity of the crises will be in proportion to the severity of your condition. If you're a two-pack-a-day smoker, for example, you'll go through more changes when you quit than if you smoke three to five cigarettes every evening.

One important thing to remember is that you may go through more than one healing crisis in your detoxification process. The body has several eliminative systems, so there will be many ways to recognize that you are moving away from the diseased condition you were living in. The healing crises are what happen to your body as it "peaks out" during the reversal or detoxification process. As your body gets closer to becoming more pure, it must go through what is considered an acute state of what had previously occurred during the worst period of the diseased condition. What this means is that for three to four days, you're going to hit a wall before you finally have a true sense of renewed health, and it usually happens as you finally believe you feel wonderful. The healing crises happen as a result of the extreme activity going on within your body, and its attempt to handle the overabundance of toxic waste. It's your body's way of dealing with the elimination of that waste.

It's important to note that nothing can bring on the "crises" except your own body saying, "It's time!" You should not fear going through such a crisis, however. In fact, it's sort of like earning a Purple Heart medal. It's earned through sacrifice and determination. (A sugar headache for two days and a stuffy "antidairy" nose for three days were part of my healing crises, but it was worth it knowing that I was finally doing something right for my body.) The crises can come in varying degrees, but rarely will your body go through more than one crisis at a time. It usually works its way through your body according to what system is being cleansed. Most healing reactions are short-lived (three to five days), though they might last a little longer, depending on how severe the damage was. The best way to get through a healing crisis (remember, this is a good thing) is to say to yourself, "I'm on a new path and I'm cleaning up my act." You have to change your old habits to change your health. Without healing there can be no cure. You get sick when your body is out of balance; when you've been doing the wrong things. Most of the time the harm is reversible, through detoxification and healing. Remember that disease (dis-ease) is nothing more than a lack of health. (Perhaps the politically correct term here would be "health-challenged.")

In the following ten chapters I'll explain the ten steps that I took to change my life and why. Read them all before deciding which step you would like to take first.

I want you to feel like a winner on this program, but remember one thing. This is not a diet. It's not some quick-weight-loss program, but rather a gradual shift in shedding your old habits (as well as pounds). Results can be dramatic in as little as two weeks, and the people who make the changes permanent never look as if they used to be heavy or unhealthy. You will have boundless energy and such an improved sense of well-being that you will carry yourself differently.

When I had my own talk show, I decided that I wanted to share this information with people all over the country. I had a forum where I could reach out to millions and provide them with the necessary information to get started. We conducted a nation-wide search for candidates who were finally ready to make this change in their lives. Narrowing down the thousands of responses to just five people was a task in itself! But we did, and one of the women we selected is now someone whom I consider not only my friend, but also my number one success story. Her name is Maggie Gillott Fountain. Maggie has lost a total of fifty-eight pounds to date, by giving up dairy and sugar, and improving the quality of her food. Today, she bears no sign that she was once heavy and unhealthy. She looks like the animal she was meant to be: a gorgeous, sleek, elegant Maggie.

> *It was a rebirth of my eating habits and my self-esteem. Here I was over 200 pounds. I wasn't looking for a quick way out. Marilu gave me the courage, the insight, to read labels and do my research. I listened to how she did it. The message is reading what you're eating—no dairy and no processed sugar. You have to be ready for it.*
>
> MAGGIE GILLOTT FOUNTAIN

> *It's a gradual process. You start by making some accommodations, and then you begin to feel better and think this isn't so bad. . . . You get purer and purer.*
>
> JOANN CARNEY, MY SISTER

❋   ❋   ❋   ❋   ❋   ❋   ❋   ❋   ❋   ❋

MAKEOVER WIMPS

For people who have a hard enough time changing their socks, let alone their lifestyle, I offer these top ten makeover tips:

1. Chemicals. Don't eat anything that glows.
2. Caffeine. No latte during *Letterman*.
3. Sugar. Don't put syrup on the *middle* pancake.
4. Meat. Switch to extra crispy, it's only 98 percent fat.
5. Dairy. Try Cheese Wiz *lite* !
6. Food combining. Never combine pickled herring with strawberry cheesecake.
7. Fat. No more Brando flicks!
8. Exercise and stress. Once a week, promise to watch someone break a sweat.
9. Sleep. Rent *Waterworld*.
10. Gusto. Try to pay more attention to beer commercials.

❋   ❋   ❋   ❋   ❋   ❋   ❋   ❋   ❋   ❋

4 | STEP 1: The Dangers of Chemicals, Additives, and Preservatives

*W*hen is food not "real" food at all? For most people, the bulk of the food they eat is filled with chemicals, preservatives, and additives, which have no nutritional value, and to put it simply, are not foods at all. Of course, all these additives are designed to do things to the food you eat, like make it look better, help it last longer, and preserve it from spoiling. Many of the foods we eat were picked, canned, or shipped a long time ago, so food manufacturers must add coloring and preservatives to keep it looking fresh. Without these additives, many of the foods we consume on a daily basis would become inedible (not to mention stink to high heaven) before they ever reached the supermarket shelves, let alone our tables. Lunch meat would turn rainbow-colored, salt would get clumpy, mayonnaise would separate and spoil, and marshmallows (now there's a "real food") would get hard as rocks.

I remember conducting experiments during chemistry class in high school. Our teacher would give us beakers full of chemicals and we would combine a few here with a few there. Imagine my surprise when my teacher told us to take a taste of these concoctions. I couldn't believe it! Peppermint! Then we mixed a few more chemicals, and before I knew it I tasted strawberry and banana! How could this be? There wasn't a "real" fruit in sight, and yet here I tasted these flavors, and they were almost as real as eating the original. The "natural strawberry" flavor actually came from bois de rose (an oil that comes from the wood of the tropical rosewood tree). I didn't think about it until years later, when I was reading about chemicals in food. Instantly, this story flashed back into my mind, and I made what I call my Helen Keller "wa wa" connection.

It all began to make sense to me. I decided right then and there that I would give up anything that wasn't a real food, anything I remembered from the Periodic Table, or anything I couldn't pronounce.

We are putting substances into our bodies that aren't meant to be there. Most of the nearly 3,000 additives used in our food are not considered harmful by the Food and Drug Administration, however, that doesn't mean that they aren't doing damage to our bodies!

Consumers need to know the facts about chemicals, food additives, and preservatives. An educated eater is a healthy eater. How does a delicious nitrate, sodium stearyl lactylate, and monocalcium phosphate sound for lunch? How about a turkey sandwich on whole wheat with potato chips? *They're often one and the same!* The FDA defines an additive as "any substance the intended use of which results or may reasonably be expected to result in affecting the characteristics of food." Chemical additives should be a frightening unknown to you. Pistachio nuts are not supposed to be red. They're red because before industrialized farming, the nut pickers would sweat and stain the nuts. The distributor had to disguise the sweat stains with red dye. Teenagers are now using the Kool-Aid we drank as kids to color their hair.

> *The average consumer eats about 140–150 pounds of food additives a year.*

Do you really know what it is you're eating? We consume these chemicals in such great amounts, there are bound to be some side effects, whether or not you are aware of them. You must learn to read labels so that you have a better understanding of what you are putting into your body. Additives can make you lethargic, sleepy, or wired, and can cause headaches and, in worst-case scenarios, cancer and other terminal diseases. Children especially, because of their low body weight, can have a reaction to these chemicals. Is it worth it?

Of course, it's not realistic to think you can live a totally preservative- or additive-free life. Chemical preservatives in food, on a global level, have been a part of our lives since World War II, when soldiers needed canned food to survive. The government knew it wasn't healthy, but it was meant to sustain life only over a short period of time. After the war, the "convenience" of canned food took the country by storm, and became a popular modern way of eating in the fifties.

You can be more aware of cutting out those chemicals that have been proven to cause major side effects as a result of ingesting them. Just because the food is sold in the local supermarket doesn't mean it's safe. Preservatives are still added for the convenience of the retailer, but not for the well-being of us, the consumers, so I personally don't want to eat anything that has a shelf life of one year (or longer). For 99 percent of the time that man has been evolving, we have only eaten food right off the tree or the vine—even refrigeration is a twentieth-century invention. I say the fresher, the better. Despite the use of modern day food additives, they are nothing new. In fact, color additives to food date back to 5000 B.C.; salt as a preservative dates back to 3000 B.C.; sulfites as a preservative can be traced to the days of ancient Rome (those Romans loved their red wine!); and herbs and spices to enhance flavor and the cosmetic look of food (often to conceal that it was spoiled) can be traced back to the biblical age.

Dangers of Food Additives and Preservatives

I have compiled a list of several common food additives found in many of the foods readily available on the shelves at your local supermarket. This list is intended to teach you what these additives and preservatives are and what they do.

Acesulfame K

Known commercially as Sunette or Sweet One, acesulfame K is a sugar substitute sold in packet or tablet form. It's used most often in chewing gum, dry mixes for beverages, instant coffee and tea, gelatin desserts, puddings, and nondairy creamers. Tests show that this additive, which has a similar chemical structure to saccharin, is known to cause cancer in animals.

Artificial Colorings

The bulk of artificial colorings used in food are synthetic dyes derived from coal tar. For decades, synthetic food dyes have been suspected of being toxic or cancer-causing, and many have been banned. (Do you remember when they had to take red M&Ms off the market because of the Red Dye #2 used to color them?) The FDA has banned thirteen synthetic food colorants since 1956 because of health concerns. Food coloring adds to the attractiveness of how a food looks. In fact, many studies over the years have shown that certain colors, such as red and black, appeal to the consumer, while other colors, such as blue, do not. I always think of the candy Chuckles and remember the red ones were always the most popular. Children's cough syrup is usually "cherry" flavored. Two of the remaining nonvegetable-based dyes on the market, Red #3 (which is used in cosmetics and to color pistachios and

49

maraschino cherries) and Yellow #5 (used in cookies, cake mixes, and soft drinks), are both linked to causing thyroid cancer in lab rats. There is no nutritional value in consuming anything that uses dye in it.

Aspartame

This sugar substitute, which is found in both Equal and Nutra-Sweet, was hailed as the great savior for dieters who went off saccharine when the FDA deemed that sugar substitute unsafe. The FDA approved the use of aspartame in 1993 for inclusion in all foods with no restrictions. This means that it can be added to foods that don't require food labeling, such as fast food. Aspartame changes into formaldehyde, phenylalanine, and methanol in the human body. It can also go through that change when a product that contains this chemical is heated to more than 86 degrees Fahrenheit. Of course, many of you might know that formaldehyde is used to preserve dead bodies. (I actually once read that embalming the human body doesn't take as long as it used to because we're halfway there already before we die.) Methanol is a deadly neurotoxin. It's believed that "Gulf War Syndrome" could be due to the heating of soft drinks that contained NutraSweet in the high temperature of the Saudi Arabian desert. There are several problems associated with aspartame, including ninety-two known side effects. One of the major problems is known as phenylketonuria (PKU). One out of 20,000 babies is born without the ability to metabolize phenylalanine, one of two amino acids found in aspartame. Toxic levels of this substance in the blood can result in mental retardation. Beyond the PKU issue, several scientists believe that aspartame might cause altered brain function and behavior changes in consumers. Some people have reported side effects such as dizziness, headaches, menstrual problems, and epileptic-like seizures after ingesting aspartame. In fact, the U.S. Air Force has warned its pilots against drinking diet soft drinks sweetened with aspartame before flying as several commercial pilots have experienced grand-mal seizures while in the cockpit. If you're pregnant, you should definitely avoid aspartame. You should also avoid giving your children this chemical because the side effects can be intensified on their little bodies.

Butylated Hydroxyanisole and Butylated Hydroxytoluene (BHA and BHT)

These two closely related chemicals are added to oil-containing foods to prevent oxidation and retard rancidity. BHA also serves as a preservative in dry foods like cereal. The International Agency for Research on Cancer (part of the World Health Organization) considers BHA and BHT carcinogenic. A 1982 study showed that BHA was linked to the growth of tumors in rats. These chemicals can accumulate in the body and cause an enlargement of the liver and slow the rate of DNA synthesis, which slows the rate of cell development. They are totally unnecessary chemical additives. To be safe, read your food labels and avoid foods that contain these potentially harmful chemicals.

Monosodium Glutamate (MSG)

Early in this century, a Japanese chemist identified MSG as the substance in certain seasonings that added to the flavor of protein-containing foods. MSG is a flavor-enhancing amino acid. Glutamine is a naturally occurring amino acid that is found in many foods, including carrots and whole grains. It is a neurotransmitter, a substance that allows cells in the brain to communicate with each other and by itself is OK. When combined with monosodium the trouble begins. Whenever I used to eat Chinese food (before I knew about MSG), I would always get a headache from it. Years later, I would discover that most Chinese food is laden with MSG, which is used to "punch up" the flavors in all the ingredients. (Accent, a popular seasoning, also has MSG in it.)

I realized that eating food that contained MSG had the same effect on me chemically as it does on food. MSG is known as an exitotoxin, which when ingested in its chemically purified form in abnormal quantities, can cause neurons in the brain to become overstimulated and die. It *always* made me feel like my brain was more sensitized. I noticed that after eating anything with MSG, I just didn't feel good. (Of course, today you can easily ask for food to be prepared without MSG.)

MSG is often disguised on processed food labels as textured vegetable protein (TVP) or plant protein extract. The word "hydrolyzed" always refers to MSG. MSG is added to frozen foods because it helps preserve the flavor. Freezing breaks down the enzymes that give fresh food its unique taste.

Common side effects associated with MSG are a tightness in the chest, drowsiness, headaches, and a burning sensation in the forearms and the back of the neck. MSG's toxicity is cumulative, so even if you don't react to it immediately, it could still be causing you problems that you're not aware of and won't be aware of for years to come.

Nitrites and Nitrates

Sodium nitrite and sodium nitrate are two closely related chemicals used to preserve cured meat, luncheon meat, ham, bacon, and hot dogs, just to name a few. While nitrates by themselves are harmless, they are easily converted to nitrites. When the nitrites combine with compounds called secondary amines, they form extremely powerful cancer-causing chemicals called nitrosamines. The chemical reaction occurs most often at high temperatures (especially when frying food). Nitrite has been linked to stomach cancer.

I remember not too long ago, I attended a conference on women's health issues. The doctor who was speaking opened the floor for a question-and-answer session. A woman raised her hand and asked the doctor, "I know nitrates are bad for my children, but how many hot dogs can I safely feed my child in a one-week period?" The doctor answered, "Eleven." I couldn't believe my ears. I fully expected him to tell the woman to stop feeding her kid hot dogs altogether, and he actually gave her "eleven" as an answer! To say that I jumped to my feet, and all over this doctor, for giving this answer is an understatement. I went off on why children shouldn't be eating anything that contains nitrites, and that there were several nitrite-free hot dogs available if your child only eats hot dogs. I also talked about the fact that foods (such as processed meats) that contain nitrates and nitrites are usually very high in fat and sodium (also things you shouldn't be feeding your kid!).

Olestra

This is the fake-fat product that was recently approved by the FDA. *Fake fat!!! Why???* Olestra was approved by our government in spite of several scientists objecting to its use. It is dangerous and unnecessary. This additive may be fat-free, but it is not fatal-free. It attaches to valuable nutrients and flushes them right out of the body. Some of these nutrients appear to protect us from such diseases as lung cancer, prostate cancer, heart disease, and macular degeneration. The Harvard School of Public Health states that "the long term consumption of olestra snack foods might therefore result in several thousand unnecessary deaths each year from lung and prostate cancers and heart disease. It is also linked to hundreds of additional cases of blindness in the elderly due to macular degeneration. Besides contributing to disease, olestra causes diarrhea and other gastrointestinal problems, even at low doses." It has also been known to cause anal leakage.

The FDA approved olestra, but all snacks containing it as an ingredient must carry a warning label that states: "This product contains olestra. Olestra may cause abdominal cramping and loose stools. Olestra inhibits the absorption of some vitamins and other nutrients. Vitamins A, D, E, and K have been added." This warning is right on the label! Why would you eat anything that makes such a strong statement about how harmful it is? Arsenic, Comet, turpentine. All poisonous. You don't consume those unless you're trying to commit suicide. Food for thought. And worst of all, I can only imagine how many overweight children will be fed olestra by well-intentioned parents, who don't realize the potential problems and embarrassment (remember anal leakage) they are causing their child.

rBGH (Recombinant Bovine Growth Hormone)

This genetically engineered drug is injected into dairy cows to increase their milk production and make them grow. It passes into the cow milk the same way pesticides pass into human milk. There are numerous issues surrounding rBGH, and the controversy over its use is growing (just like the cows). It's hard to understand why dairy farmers are justified in using this chemical when there is actually a milk surplus in this country, and the government uses your tax dollars to purchase the excess milk from dairy farmers whether it gets used or not.

   This chemical has been linked to cancer. It also causes diseases in cows that require excessive amounts of antibiotics to be used to treat the disease. Of course, those antibiotics are passed on to us with every slice of cheese, glass of milk, spoonful of yogurt, or pat of butter we consume.

Saccharin

Several studies conducted in the 1970s linked saccharin with cancer in lab animals. Saccharin contains the same type of warning as olestra. You should simply avoid consuming anything that contains saccharin.

Sulfites

Sulfites are a class of synthetically produced chemicals that keep cut fruits and vegetables looking fresh. They also prevent discoloration in apricots, raisins, and other dried fruits, as well as processed seafood, dehydrated soup mixes, and syrups. They control and prevent discoloration, bacterial growth, and fermentation in wine. Until the early 1980s, they were considered safe, but there have been six scientific studies proving that sulfites can provoke severe allergic reactions. In 1985, the FDA identified at least a dozen deaths linked to sulfites (all those deaths were linked to people with asthma). In that same year, Congress finally forced the FDA to ban sulfites from most fruits and vegetables. The FDA ban does not cover fresh-cut potatoes, dried fruits, and wine, so if you're asthmatic, you should avoid those foods. Sulfites are still commonly (and illegally) used in restaurant salad bars to preserve the raw vegetables.

Obviously, if you suffer from any of the noted side effects from the ingestion and consumption of these chemicals, you don't need a study to tell you that you should stop eating them. But you might not know you're suffering from the side effects until it's too late. There's also a cumulative effect that is taking place. In the face of making a choice for your health, experts all agree that you must weigh the risks versus the benefits when it comes to chemicals. For some, the benefits are the convenience, economic value, and protection against food-borne disease-producing agents. The risks, however, seem to outweigh the long-term effects of most of these benefits. A safe plan of action is to avoid consuming large amounts of any of these additives. Choose to eat a diet that consists of natural foods made by God rather than a chemist.

Organic Food

The preservation as well as the presentation of food is a business like any other business. It's based on turning a profit. If the food lasts longer or looks more attractive because it's been "doctored," people buy the products.

In recent months, there has been quite a bit of controversy surrounding the FDA setting a standard definition of what is an "organic" food. To date, seventeen states have various guidelines that qualify a food as "organic." "Organic" is not a type of food but a method of producing foods without using synthetic fertilizers and pesticides. The organic food industry saw $3.5 billion in sales in 1996, and at least 50 percent of the supermarkets in America now have an "organic food" section. Buying a product that says "certified organic" is the best insurance that you are getting a truly organic product. This means that the farmer's crops were grown in soil that has been free of prohibited synthetic pesticides for at least three years. It also means that the farmer is actively nurturing additional land so it will be fertile and plentiful for future generations' food needs. Processed foods that meet the requirements can also be labeled as organic. At least 95 percent of the ingredients have to be grown and processed according to the standards to earn that label. Additives, such as artificial preservatives, dyes, and flavorings, are absolutely forbidden.

Until recently, organic meat was an oxymoron. Today, you can get organic meats, which means the livestock was raised on only organic feed, without growth hormones or antibiotics, and were treated humanely, being allowed to roam freely through the pastures and barnyards where they were raised. (This is also associated with free-range products.) I remember introducing my family to "organic" turkey during Thanksgiving 1979. It was by far the best turkey we had ever tasted (and the first turkey I ever bought that didn't come with a little pop-up thermometer!).

The question I am asked most frequently on this topic is whether organic food is better than nonorganic food. As I have said many times throughout this book, improve the quality of your food, and you will improve the quality of your health. Sometimes organic foods aren't as appealing to the eye, but their flavors are plentiful. Without all the preservatives and additives, the shelf life of certain produce is shortened. Nutritionally speaking, without a doubt, the lack of all those additives makes organic food better for you.

Fear of pesticides seems to be the reason that the demand for organic food is skyrocketing. Chemicals such as DDT have been proven dangerous enough to be banned from the United States. The use of pesticides in farming has been linked to immune system diseases, nerve damage, and disruptions in the endocrine system, which regulates hormones and fertility. Other chemicals ruin the topsoil used to farm and run into the water supply on the property as well. That water is used to keep the already tainted topsoil moist and to satiate the animals' thirst. In addition, many farms, which raise cattle as well as farm produce, do not have enough distance between where the cows (and other farm animals) eliminate body waste and where the water supply is contained. Animal feces are the biggest cause of *E. coli* poisoning. In 1997, a four-year-old girl from California ate *E. coli* tainted packaged lettuce. An investigation revealed that the water supply used to wash the lettuce prior to its being packaged and shipped to the store for consumption was infested with these deadly bacteria. This poor little girl will now have lifelong kidney and vision problems after suffering through a fourteen-week stay in the hospital. Although the Centers for Disease Control and the FDA are getting better at identifying and correcting these problems, as long as animals live on farms where vegetation is grown, these problems will persist.

Nine thousand Americans die from tainted food each year.

Until federal regulators implement national standards on organic foods and reassess the use of pesticides on crops, you should always wash all produce in water before eating it. Pesticide experts estimate that at least 25–50 percent of the residue is removed. Limit your consumption of imported fruits and vegetables unless they have been certified as organic. Imported foods have a higher rate of pesticide residue and are more likely to harbor dangerous microbes and parasites. Don't assume that organic food is truly organic unless it has been certified.

5 | STEP 2: Caffeine and Nicotine— Breaking the Habit

What drug do four out of five Americans take on any given day? How about caffeine! It's found in coffee, tea, chocolate, cocoa, soft drinks, aspirin, and some analgesics commonly used for pain relief.

A Stimulating Brew

Caffeine is in fact a drug, and can be highly addictive. It doesn't take much to develop a dependency on this drug, as it is so readily available and is an ingredient in many foods and drinks consumed every day. There are brand-name products such as Surge, Jolt, Aqua Buzz, and Krank20 that sound more like street names for hard-core drugs than names for soft drinks, but they are in fact the names of caffeine-spiked beverages. Caffeine is the most overused stimulant in the world. It is considered a stimulant and it affects the nervous system. It is a drug that artificially elevates your mood and supposedly fights fatigue. Recent studies, however, show that caffeine can actually pose significant health risks, especially for unsuspecting susceptible people. It can cause hypertension, abnormal heart rhythms, problems with pregnancy and birth, osteoporosis, ulcers, and heartburn, as well as panic and anxiety attacks. An overdose of caffeine can overstimulate your nerves, making you feel anxious, jittery, irritable, and even cause you to tremble. Too much caffeine can cause diarrhea and hot flashes.

I remember the first time I ever tried coffee, at age fifteen. I drank two sips, and I felt nervous. I started to shake, I felt sick to my stomach, and I even started to sweat! This was from two little sips! Do you remember the first time you drank a cup of coffee? How did you feel? That reaction is still happening to you every time you drink a cup of coffee. We've become so desensitized to caffeine and its effects, we don't even notice. Try giving up caffeine for three weeks and then have just one cup of coffee. You will feel panicky, jittery, and your heart will race. Can you imagine the toll it takes on your body over years of abuse? We have to ease up on the consumption to help eliminate long-term damage.

Eight ounces of Dannon Coffee Yogurt packs the same caffeine punch as a twelve-ounce can of Coke.

So what exactly is caffeine? Well, it's similar in structure to adenosine, which is a chemical found in the brain that actually slows down its activity. Since the two chemicals compete with each other, the more caffeine you consume, the less adenosine becomes available. That explains why caffeine can temporarily heighten concentration and keep you from being sleepy. Within thirty to sixty minutes of drinking a cup of coffee, for example, caffeine will reach its peak penetration in the bloodstream. It typically takes four to six hours for those effects to wear off. Interestingly, coffee accounts for only three-quarters of the daily caffeine intake Americans consume. Tea, soft drinks, and chocolate make up most of the remaining 25 percent.

Caffeine Overload

There's the good, the bad, and the ugly when it comes to caffeine. While it is true that you can get a quick jolt of energy from drinking a cup of coffee, it doesn't last very long, and often you'll find yourself jittery and nervous from the caffeine. If you drink too much caffeine, you can find yourself unable to fall asleep. It can overstimulate the nerves, making you feel restless, anxious, nervous, and irritable. The amount of caffeine needed to trigger a reaction depends on your own sensitivity to the drug and how often you drink it. The reason we drink caffeine in the first place is because we love the rush of energy and temporary euphoria we get from it. However, because our bodies become desensitized to caffeine so quickly, we must continually increase our daily dosage if we still want to achieve that energy rush. Eventually, we need a huge daily dose just to feel normal, That normalcy involves a lot of energy ups and downs throughout the day, which is a common pattern for most drugs that are addictive. Some people are so desensitized to caffeine, they can drink a strong cup of coffee just before going to bed. Some people suffer very few side effects from caffeine, while others, especially if they're not used to it, can have a major reaction from the slightest amount. (I can get a headache from just walking by a Starbucks!) Caffeine can also cause facial flushing, diarrhea, and frequent urination. People with high blood pressure should avoid caffeine altogether, because it can raise blood pressure.

There is some research that shows consuming caffeine has a few benefits. Caffeine in moderation can fight drowsiness, fatigue, and muscular fatigue, and improve your mood and performance. The key word here is "moderation," because most people use caffeine in excess. It doesn't take much to develop a dependency on caffeine, either. One study shows that one to three cups of coffee a day will do it. The average cup of coffee (six ounces) typically supplies around 100 milligrams of caffeine. It can vary, depending on how the coffee is prepared. The more coffee grounds you use, how fine they were ground, and the longer you brew the coffee, the more caffeine there will be. The average adult consumes around 200 milligrams of caffeine a day, and the top percentage of those people take in more than 400 milligrams a day! Drinking more than 600 milligrams a day can lead to stomach ulcers, hand tremors, an irregular heartbeat, and insomnia. Caffeine promotes stomach acid secretion, so it can be a potentially dangerous substance for those with peptic ulcers.

Are You a Java Junkie?

How do you know if you're dependent on caffeine? Try eliminating all caffeine from your diet for three days. See how you feel. If you get a throbbing headache, you're probably drinking too much caffeine. The amount of withdrawal is usually equal to the amount of addiction. Quitting caffeine can have some pretty significant side effects. The most common complaint is a frequent headache. One study showed that 10 percent of those who quit caffeine went through severe withdrawal symptoms. They became depressed and fatigued, and some even complained of flulike symptoms, including nausea and vomiting. In general, the symptoms appear within twelve to twenty-four hours after kicking the habit, and virtually all caffeine in your body is eliminated during that time. The withdrawal symptoms seem to be the worst on the first or second day and can last up to a week, although the usual time is four days.

You can quit cold turkey or gradually wean yourself off caffeine. You have to decide what you can handle. If you drink coffee only in the morning, the craving you have first thing in the morning for that cup of joe may actually be a withdrawal symptom. Sometimes people drink coffee only during the week, so on the weekends, they might suffer some withdrawal-like symptoms.

But coffee, although the most common source of caffeine, isn't the only culprit. Two to four cans of caffeinated soda or two to four cups of tea can provide as much caffeine as a cup or two of coffee. A cup of black tea (it's the most common tea in America) supplies around fifty milligrams of caffeine. Green tea and oolong tea have much less caffeine, and herbal teas don't have any. Seventy-five percent of the caffeine contained in tea seeps through the tea in the first thirty seconds of brewing. Furthermore, eight of the ten best-selling brands of soda contain caffeine. Most of these contain thirty-five to forty-five milligrams of caffeine, but some are much higher. The kola nut extract used to flavor colas naturally contains caffeine. Manufacturers say that they add caffeine to balance out the sweetness, but the real reason is to keep you drinking their products. Chocolate contains caffeine because the cocoa bean powder used to make the candy contains natural caffeine. An average chocolate bar contains around thirty milligrams. One of the most surprising sources of hidden caffeine is everyday medications. Manufacturers can add as much as 100 milligrams of caffeine to certain cold medicines, muscle relaxers, pain relievers, and antimigraine drugs. So if you're popping back a couple of aspirin every four hours, you could be taking in a hefty dose of caffeine in the process. Read your product labels! Stay away from over-the-counter stimulants that are supposed to keep you up, because they're loaded with caffeine.

Certain drugs that you might be taking can interfere with, slow down, or prevent your body from ridding itself of caffeine. Birth control pills, certain heart medications containing verapamil, and the ulcer drug cimetidine can all have this adverse affect. Likewise, drugs that stimulate the nervous system, including appetite suppressants, asthma medications, oral decongestants, and thyroid hormones also have adverse side effects when combined with caffeine. They can cause insomnia, irritability, nervousness, and heart palpitations. Tranquilizers and antidepressants also don't mix well with caffeine. The combination can result in severe hypertension and abnormal heart rhythms.

Caffeine Health Risks

Over the past several years, caffeine has been linked to an added risk of cancer, coronary heart disease, osteoporosis, hypertension, and even prenatal problems. The risks are individual depending on your genetic predisposition toward developing these diseases. Your tolerance to caffeine depends on the genetic makeup of the liver enzymes, which help eliminate caffeine from the body.

It's not easy to get a handle on caffeine and its connection to health because we rarely consume caffeine by itself. It's always mixed with something else, including lots of other chemicals. In general, people who drink coffee tend to also be smokers, eat a fattier diet, and/or drink alcohol. They are less likely to take good care of themselves than people who drink decaffeinated beverages are. Studies show that those who drink caffeine-free beverages are more likely to take vitamins, exercise regularly, and eat a centered diet. They're even more likely to wear their seat belts while driving! (If you do drink decaffeinated beverages, be aware of how the caffeine was taken out. It's better to use water-pressed decaffeinated coffee than to use a coffee where the caffeine is bleached out by chemicals. So make sure the label says "water-pressed.")

According to a recent study of 233 surgery patients, regular caffeine drinkers are three times more likely to wind up with a postoperative headache than those who do not drink caffeine.

The fact that many chemically dependent people are also heavy consumers of coffee is no great shock. Caffeine and cigarettes usually replace the previously abused substances. Developing a dependency on caffeine is especially unhealthy for these people.

A dose of caffeine can raise blood pressure in people who are occasional caffeine drinkers. Drinking anything that contains caffeine before working out is never a good idea because it can elevate your blood pressure even more than usual and sometimes to a near-dangerous level for those with hypertension. People who experience palpitations from caffeine should avoid consuming anything that contains the drug.

If you're trying to get pregnant, you'd better cut the caffeine out of your diet. Several studies have shown that caffeine can impair fertility, especially if you have three or more cups of coffee (or the equivalent in other products) worth of caffeine a day. Pregnant women eliminate caffeine from their body more slowly than usual. The caffeine can reach the fetus, which also has difficulty eliminating caffeine. The fetus can get overstimulated, have abnormal heart rhythms, and get the jitters before and after birth as a result. Heavy caffeine consumption during pregnancy is not a good idea, and it should be avoided. After pregnancy, a nursing mother can pass on caffeine to the baby through her milk, causing insomnialike symptoms for the child. (Not a good thing for Mommy or the baby!)

Caffeine can also be hard on your bones. The more caffeine a woman drinks, the more calcium she excretes in her urine. She is losing an extra five milligrams of calcium for every six ounces of coffee (one cup) or two cans of soda. The FDA banned the use of caffeine in over-the-counter weight-loss drugs in 1991 (caffeine has no long-term effect on weight). It is still used in aspirin and other painkillers, however. Caffeine increases their potency by 40 percent.

Caffeine is found in so many different products that merely switching to decaffeinated coffee won't solve the problem for you, but it will help reduce your intake if you can't bear the thought of leading a coffee-less life. Read nutritional labels on everything and go for the brands that are caffeine-free whenever possible. If you do decide to eliminate caffeine from your life, back off it slowly if you start to get headaches. You will win the battle of the bean if you stick with it.

Smoking

People who smoke telegraph to the world that they have problems. With everything we know about smoking today, if you can't quit something that is obviously dangerous to your health and to the people around you, then you probably have psychological problems that are holding you back from living a healthy life. I was a pack-a-day smoker from 1971 to 1979. It started when I couldn't lose the weight I had put on the summer of 1970. I had gained so much weight that my mother actually suggested to me that I take up smoking to help me lose the excess pounds!

Women who smoke are twice as likely to suffer a stroke and three times as likely to suffer from heart disease as nonsmoking women.

(She smoked two or three cigarettes a night after dinner.) I hated the taste of the smoke so much that I wound up eating to disguise the bad aftertaste.

I smoked in college, and I would go through phases of thinking, "I'm a smoker, I should be smoking!" Ultimately, I smoked about a pack a day before I gave it up for good. I decided to quit because I knew it wasn't good for me, and I really wanted my sister to quit, too; she was up to almost three packs a day!

There's so much information regarding the dangers to your health if you smoke. The bottom line is that you are inhaling pure chemicals and doing long-term damage to your body, your skin, and your health. In addition to nicotine, cigarette smoke contains around 4,000 chemicals. Some chemicals are poisons, like arsenic, formaldehyde, and DDT. Your lungs retain about 90 percent of these compounds and pass them into your bloodstream. Nicotine in the tobacco causes the adrenal glands to secrete hormones that increase blood pressure and heart rate, causing your heart to work extra hard.

If you're afraid of gaining weight when you quit smoking, don't be. According to the CDC, a recent study shows that the average weight gain for people who stop smoking is only five pounds. The weight gain can be easily managed through careful diet and stress management. Their study even showed that a great number of people *lose* weight when they quit smoking. It's a choice to get healthy, not a ticket to eat. It is possible to lose weight and not smoke at the same time. Studies have shown that smokers feel as if they have less control over their lives than nonsmokers do. That's why non-smokers (not at first, but eventually) have a much easier time controlling their weight. In general, they take more pride in their lives.

> *One out of every five people dies from a smoking-related disease each year worldwide.*

If smoking doesn't kill you, it will make you old before your time. Nothing ages you more than smoking does. On the average, smokers tend to look five to ten years older than their actual ages because of the wrinkles around their eyes and mouths caused from inhaling. Smoking damages the elastic tissue that keeps skin tight. If you want to slow down the aging process, don't smoke.

Besides, smoking stinks!

6 | STEP 3: The Not-So-Sweet Bad News About Sugar and Aspartame

I was a kid with a real sweet tooth. I loved anything that was sugary. Even as a child, I recognized that once I ate sugar for breakfast, I wanted it all day long. But getting caught up on that sugar treadmill is dangerous, *especially* for children. When I was shopping in New York recently with my husband, we were at the counter of a lighting store waiting to pay for our purchase. I remember catching sight of an adorable little girl out of the corner of my eye. She was so calm and well-behaved. There was a candy dish on the counter, and she asked her parents if she could take a piece of

> **Sugar:** *Refined sucrose, produced by multiple chemical processing of the juice of the sugar cane beet and removal of all fiber and protein, which amount to 90 percent of the natural plant.*

candy. Her mother agreed, and she gobbled it down. A few minutes later, I noticed this child had gone from being sweet and calm to being a little jittery and nervous. She started to ask if she could have another piece of candy, and her mother said, "In a little while." As each second passed, this little girl got more and more agitated and impatient, repeating her query, "Now can I?" "Now can I?" "Now can I?" Eventually, she became totally overwhelmed and consumed by her sugar fix, twitching and tapping her feet relentlessly.

I have often referred to sugar as "kiddy cocaine," because in my opinion, that is exactly what it is. Watching your child's behavior change right before your very eyes from eating sugar can be a very dramatic experience. Giving children sugar is like giving them a drug: It stimulates, causes mood swings, and can be addicting. Sugar is an unhealthy food choice and it overstimulates kids, making them unruly.

> *Americans consume somewhere in the neighborhood of 136 pounds of sugar per person, per year.*

Sugar adds calories to your daily intake, and those are often "empty" (meaning no nutritional value) calories. Over half the sugar consumed today is added directly from the sugar bowl while eating or preparing a meal. The food manufacturers add the other half, either as sugar or as high-fructose corn syrup. Your body breaks down sugar that you eat into the sugar found in the blood, called glucose.

Sugar phobia has risen to an all-time high in recent years (and for good reason), with refined white sugar being blamed for hyperactivity, diabetes, hypoglycemia, bad moods, yeast infections, obesity, and tooth decay. Food manufacturers have cashed in on this panic by offering substitute products that contain honey, fruit juice, and other sweeteners that are considered healthier. The key thing to understand is that many of these substitutes *could* contain as much sugar as refined white sugar products, or they might be chemically manufactured synthetic sweeteners (aspartame, acesulfame K, saccharin) that pose major health concerns.

Refined white sugar depletes your body of all the B vitamins. It leaches calcium from your hair, blood, bones, and teeth. It interferes with the absorption of calcium, protein, and other minerals in your body, and retards the growth of valuable intestinal bacteria. White sugar is a simple carbohydrate made up of two simple sugars, fructose and glucose. Those two elements are also found in natural sugars such as honey, corn syrup, brown sugar, and concentrated fruit juice sweeteners. Natural sugar is found in a lot of foods, too, such as grains, fruits, vegetables, and other complex carbohydrates, which end up as glucose in the blood after your body has extracted the essential vitamins, minerals, and fiber the natural sugar is packed with.

Sugar ferments in your stomach. It stops the secretion of gastric juices and inhibits the stomach's ability to digest. Sugar is not partially digested in the mouth by saliva as other foods are. When eaten alone, it passes directly into the small intestine, but when eaten with other foods, they get stuck in the stomach for a while. The warm and moist conditions of the stomach guarantee rapid acid fermentation. So drinking a regular soda with your meal or sugar in your coffee while eating breakfast definitely ignites that fire.

> *The first thing I gave up was sugar. It seemed like the easiest of Marilu's ten steps for me to try. I couldn't believe the difference in my energy level. Marilu said to me, "Just try one step at a time," and so I made my first step sugar. I'm very enthusiastic about my results.*
> LILLIE KAE STEVENS,
> PERFORMER IN BROADWAY MUSICAL *CHICAGO*

Get off the Sugar Treadmill

Kicking the sugar habit isn't an easy thing to do. I know that giving up refined sugar was a difficult decision for me. I remember someone once told me that refined sugar is so addictive, you can eat a pound of chocolate but you can't eat a pound of dates. It made me laugh, because I thought, "I'm going to try this and see if I can eat a pound of dates *and* a pound of chocolate." (Not at the same time, however.) You know what? I couldn't do it. The pound of chocolate was so easy for me to eat, I could have eaten more. But sure enough, that pound of dates wasn't happening. (And I love dates!) My theory on this one is that once you start eating refined sugar, you want more and more of it, even if your stomach tells you it's full. (That's the sugar treadmill.) The dates satisfy that "something sweet" urge you're having because they're a naturally sweet whole food. The chocolate has more of a chemical effect, because the refined sugar is so addictive. It goes beyond satisfying a simple urge. People generally eat to fill their stomachs, not caring what they put into it. But you should care, because so much of how we feel and think and act are all tied to what we eat.

The brain depends on blood glucose for its energy. Eating sucrose can cause a wide variety of blood glucose levels. I remember reading that a lawyer tried to get his criminal client off the hook by using his "high-sugar" junk food diet, notably Twinkies, as his defense for his irrational behavior; the lawyer claimed the junk food made the defendant hypoglycemic! This is another case of extreme food causing extreme behavior (or exploitation of the law—you decide).

If you want to get off that sugar treadmill, try cutting down on your total sugar intake. Eliminate all added sugars, and decrease your intake of foods that are high in refined sugar. It's that simple.

I found that when I gave up sugar, I also ended up giving up red meat. They are total opposites in terms of being yin (sugar) and yang (meat). The reason you crave one with the other is that they balance each other out because they're both so extreme on the food number line. Dropping both from your diet makes it easier to stick with not eating either food because your craving for both goes way down. The more vegetable protein you eat in place of animal protein, the lower your desire for sugar will be. That taste for something sweet after you eat simply fades after a while because you're eating a much more balanced meal.

Once you decide to kick the sugar habit, you'll notice that your taste buds will start picking up flavors and sensations you may have never experienced before. Everything you eat will start to taste better and more alive in its flavor. Oddly enough, it's not only the food that tastes better, it's your body that's better able to taste the food. (You'll find that this is a common side effect when choosing any one of my ten steps.)

Sugar Substitutes

My intent in encouraging you to give up sugar is not to take the sweet temptation out of your life, but rather to improve the quality of your health and food choices. If you're ready to take refined sugar out of your diet, I suggest clearing out all the food items in your home that might be a temptation. Get rid of the candy bars, the cookies, and the ice cream. Here's the good news: You can get sweet substitutes for practically every item in your cupboards, refrigerator, and freezer. If you drink coffee with sugar and/or milk, my suggestion is to get rid of all three things. But I know some of you are very attached to that cup of joe, so try using raw honey as a sweetener. Better yet, use Rice Dream rice milk, which is slightly sweet. You could always switch to flavored herbal tea, which is easy to drink without any added sweetener.

Brown Sugar

Brown sugar is often suggested as a sugar substitute, but in reality brown sugar is white sugar with a dye job! Molasses is added to refined sugar, and that is what makes the sugar brown. The rawlike illusion is a result of a specially designed crystallization process that is strictly for aesthetics.

Saccharin

Several studies conducted in the 1970s linked saccharin with cancer in lab animals. Saccharin contains the same type of warning as olestra. You should avoid consuming anything that contains saccharin.

Aspartame

Aspartame, which is found in both Equal and NutraSweet, was hailed as the great savior for dieters who went off saccharin when the FDA deemed that sugar substitute unsafe. The FDA approved the use of aspartame in 1993 for inclusion in all foods with no restrictions. This means that it can be added to foods that don't require food labeling, such as fast food. Some people have reported side effects such as dizziness, headaches, menstrual problems, and epileptic-like seizures after ingesting aspartame. There have also been studies that link the use of aspartame to causing an increase in cell mutation, possibly resulting in brain tumors.

Because of their lower body weight, children consuming adult-size quantities of this sweetener have much higher blood concentrations of aspartame. As few as five servings a day can impair brain function in a fifty-pound child.

Another concern with aspartame is that it has no nutritional value. Most people use it because it's low in calories, but this choice cancels out using a sweetener that might have needed nutrients, like raw honey or fruit juice sweeteners. For the record, one package of Equal has around four calories and less than one gram of carbohydrates. That tiny package is equivalent to two teaspoons of sugar. The American Dietetic Association has expressed great concern about aspartame, saying that even though studies support its safety, they still do not know what the long-term effects will be. For more information on aspartame, see Chapter 4.

Acesulfame K

Known commercially as Sunette or Sweet One, acesulfame (acesulfame K) is a sugar substitute sold in packet or tablet form. It's used most often in chewing gum, dry mixes for beverages, instant coffee and tea, gelatin desserts, puddings, and nondairy creamers. Tests show that this additive, which has a chemical structure similar to that of saccharin, is known to cause cancer in animals.

Honey

Replacing refined sugar with raw honey is a good idea, but be aware that honey is more concentrated than white sugar. You need to use only half the amount of honey as you would sugar. Honey is assimilated into the bloodstream very quickly, and it has certain minerals and enzymes that don't upset the body's mineral balance as much as sugar does.

Honey was used as medicine for centuries. It has natural properties that can have a healing effect on the liver, neutralize toxins in the body, and even work as a pain reliever. If you eat a mostly grain and vegetable diet, a small amount of honey is usually enough to satisfy your taste needs.

Because honey is so concentrated, you might consider diluting it with water before you use it. If you use honey, go for raw, completely unprocessed, unheated honey.

Sucrose and Fructose

Sucrose and fructose are often used in combination as a sugar substitute, though they are both sugars. Sucrose has little negative effect on the body, but an excessive amount might upset the blood-sugar balance. Fructose, which is substantially sweeter than white sugar, does not overtax the pancreas to make insulin as refined sugar does.

Maltose

The least concentrated, least sweet, and the closest to being whole-food sugar substitutes are products that contain maltose. They are one-third as sweet as white sugar and are not highly processed. Rice syrup and barley malt are primarily maltose and are very easy to find in health food stores. One of the main reasons I recommend these as excellent substitutes is that at least half of the composition of the grain-based sweeteners are nutrients found in whole grains. They also take longer to digest in the stomach.

That helps even out blood-sugar peaks and valleys that highly refined sugar can cause. If you've never tried rice syrup or barley malt, I highly recommend that you give them a try. They're really tasty, easy to use in recipes, and extremely easy to get used to.

Cane Juice

For those of you who have become so used to sprinkling a spoonful of sugar on your cereal or in your morning coffee, a relatively healthy substitution is unrefined, granulated cane juice. (It has been around for over 5,000 years in some parts of the world!) It's made by evaporating the water from whole sugar cane juice. This sugar has a lot more nutrients and mineralization to help prevent tooth decay and the other diseases often brought on by refined white sugar. Read your food labels. Anything that reads "dried cane juice" or "cane juice" is based with this substitute.

Lactose and Fruit Juice Sweeteners

It's not a good idea to use lactose (from milk) because it contains a sugar component called galactose that is sometimes difficult for people to digest. Fruit juices are an excellent replacement because they're easily available and are relatively low in sweetness. When they are used in fruit syrups, their sugar content is much higher.

Remember that when you are using sugar substitutes, they are often sweeter than refined sugar, so you don't need as much of them. Until you have weaned yourself off the bad sugar and cleaned out your system a little, your body may be confused and continue to respond as though it were still getting the bad stuff. Cut back on sweets and neutralize your palate a little before really going gung-ho with all these substitutes.

CHEMICALLY PROCESSED SWEETENERS

Sweetener	Source
White sugar	Cane and sugar beets
Raw sugar	Cane and sugar beets
Brown sugar	White sugar with molasses added
Corn syrup	Processed from corn starch
Blackstrap molasses	By-product of granulated sugar (contains minerals)

Fructose, xylitol, and sorbitol can be made from natural sources, but it is too expensive, so they are refined from commercial glucose and sucrose.

NATURALLY PROCESSED SWEETENERS

Sweetener	Composition Source
Unrefined sugar	Unrefined cane juice powder
Maple syrup	Boiled-down sugar maple tree sap
Sorghum molasses	Cooked-down cane juice
Barbados molasses	Cooked-down cane juice
Rice syrup and barley malt	Fermented grains—less destructive to the body's mineral balance
Honey	Nectar from flowers processed in the stomach of bees
Fruit juices	Fruit
Fruit syrups and date sugar	Fruit—far more concentrated and sweeter than fresh fruit
Amasake	Fermented rice maltose

The Scoop on Sugar

Eating a diet laden with lots of excess sugar will surely take a toll on your body and your health. The evidence of the damage sugar can do is best displayed by tooth decay. Certain bacteria in the mouth break down the sugar that remains after eating, which produces an acid that can erode the enamel on your teeth. This bacteria feed off any kind of sugar, so sugar that is produced by breaking down starchy foods can be just as bad as drinking a soda or eating a candy bar when it comes to decay. The key to keeping your mouth healthy is good oral hygiene. Children need to be especially tuned in to taking good care of their teeth, since they usually eat a lot of sugar. Making sure they (and you) brush with fluoride toothpaste and floss regularly will remove the sugar-induced bacteria.

Sugar may be a major reason so many Americans are overweight these days. Fat is the main culprit, but why are so many people gaining weight eating low-fat and even no-fat snacks? People think these low-fat food choices are a ticket to eat twice as much food, and they forget that low-fat and no-fat don't necessarily mean no calories or sugar. If you want to lose weight and keep it off, you must cut down on fat and sugar to see results. (Good thing they're two of my steps, huh?)

Diabetics have been told to stay away from sugar and sugary foods because they can cause a surge in their already high blood glucose levels. The truth is that diabetics must eat a balanced meal that includes some protein and fat. Sugar in moderation for most is all right, but whenever possible, it ought to be substituted with another carbohydrate that doesn't have any measurable sugar.

The diagnosis of hypoglycemia (low blood-sugar levels) may result from intestinal, kidney, and liver abnormalities, and other conditions that might interfere with the body's normally tight regulation of blood sugar. The symptoms are often misdiagnosed because they are so common to other ailments. They include sweating, anxiety, hunger, and weakness.

Sugar plays a major role in altering one's mood, but after the positive stimulation comes the sugar crash, a severe opposite reaction. Someone who eats a candy bar, drinks a soda, or eats a sugary pastry may feel a temporary energy lift, but soon thereafter, feels tired, nervous, irritable, and often depressed. Refined sugar has a chemical reaction on the brain, releasing the "feel good" hormone serotonin, tricking the body into a temporary lift and an increase in blood-sugar levels, too. (It's believed that carbohydrates have the same effect, so if you need that lift, you don't have to get it from sugar.)

Refined sugar is believed to cause hyperactivity, especially in children. It reacts in the body, which then releases adrenaline into the bloodstream, resulting in feelings of anxiety, excitement, and problems with concentrating. I believe that many of the children being diagnosed with Attention Deficit Disorder, Attention Deficit Hyperactive Disorder, and Learning Deficit Disorder may just be reacting to sugar, or their sugar reactions are making the disorder even worse. I think it is wise for the children who suffer from these disorders to have their sugar intake monitored.

Some children have other intolerances to sugar. Galactosemia (an intolerance to the sugar component of lactose) affects one in every 30,000 to 60,000 infants. It's similar to having a lactose intolerance, but with symptoms that are far more severe, especially in infants. If galactosemia goes untreated after birth, the child may suffer from stunted growth, cataracts, liver disorders, or even death. Mild symptoms can cause a baby to vomit, lose weight, and become lethargic. Outside of dairy products, the probable cause of galactosemia is the consumption of foods high in galactose levels, such as tomato, apple sauce, squash, watermelon, papaya, and persimmon. Bananas, apples, dates, kiwis, pumpkin, bell peppers, and brussels sprouts have a moderate level of galactose.

Government studies show that American adults get an average of 20 percent of their calories from sugar. That's around 25 teaspoons of sugar a day! Children are eating even more than that. That's way too much consumption of empty calories that provide no nutrients. When you do eat sugar, it should be from a natural source, such as fruit. One thing is certain: We eat too much sugar for our own good.

7 | STEP 4: The Health Risks of Meat

*A*fter my mother died, I started thinking a lot about everything related to my health and my eating. I began to think about the way that animals are slaughtered, and I remember someone once told me a story that right before an animal is killed, it gets a rush of adrenaline through its body. That adrenaline gets trapped in its veins and muscles, and that is what we eat when we eat its flesh. As when I gave up Tab, I figured that I would try to give up meat (beef, pork, lamb) for three weeks. If I didn't feel any different after the initial three weeks, I would go back to eating it. Fortunately for me, I never went back. Obviously, the beef farmers aren't going to be too happy with me on this, but I do not consider meat an essential food group.

Before 1979, I used to love meat, especially rare roast beef. I ate bacon, sausage, pastrami, steak. You name it, if it was red and rare, I ate it. The last time I ate meat was when I went to visit John Travolta (my boyfriend at the time) on the set of *Urban Cowboy*. I went out to pick up some of our favorite foods from a local deli for lunch. I looked at the counter and saw some juicy rare roast beef. On my way back to meet John, I rolled up a piece and popped it into my mouth. It tasted terrible. It had been four months since I had eaten meat, and suddenly I could see the marbleized fat, and realized I was eating the flesh of another animal. It seemed so wrong and it didn't taste anything like I had remembered.

Humans were meant to be vegetarians. Our closest living relatives from the animal world, apes, are 98 percent vegetarians. Even cows are, by nature, vegetarians. (We're just getting their healthy grass and grain diet once removed!) The structure of our skin, teeth, stomach, and bowels, and the length of our digestive system, are all typical of vegetarian animals. Somewhere along the way, we overcame our physical limitations and decided to kill other animals for food. If you took away all modern technology, which slaughters, butchers, and delivers meat to our local grocery stores, the shelves would be filled with nothing but fruits, vegetables, and grains—the foods God intended for us to eat. Of course, you can survive quite easily on a diet that consists of no animal products whatsoever, often referred to as a vegan diet.

Most of the world's human population is largely vegetarian. Despite the information that is put out by the Meat and Livestock Commission, humans do not need meat. People always say, "I don't feel strong when I don't eat meat. Meat gives me strength." The largest, strongest dinosaur, the brontosaurus, was a vegetarian. An elephant is a vegetarian. Eating meat has nothing to do with strength. In fact, it zaps your strength because it overtaxes your digestive system and wears you out. Eating meat, especially red meat, is associated with promoting your risk of cancer. People who eat red meat five or more times a week

> *Some 100,000 cows die each year from disease. These diseased cows are ground up and fed to other cows—cows that we eat.*

are four times more likely to have colon cancer than people who eat no meat or eat meat less than once a month. Prostate cancer is another risk, and women who eat beef, lamb, or pork as a daily main dish are two and a half times more likely to develop colon cancer than women who eat meat less than once a month. The substitution of other protein sources such as beans and lentils is known to reduce the risk of colon cancer.

Meats are high in animal fat, which are hard for us to digest and therefore stay in our bodies for a long time. The human digestive system wasn't meant to break down the flesh from another animal.

Seeing Red—
How Animals Are Slaughtered

The Pure Food and Drug Act of 1906 requires, for sanitary reasons, that no slaughtered animal may fall into the blood of another slaughtered animal. Animals being slaughtered in the United States are shackled around the rear legs and hoisted into the air. They hang by one leg, fully conscious, upside down on a conveyer belt for between two and five minutes (sometimes even longer) before the slaughterer can make his cut. How these animals suffer! The cows are exhausted and terrified, until they are provoked into hysteria. They hang upside down and twist frantically, sometimes rupturing joints or breaking a leg, in terrible pain and terror. If slaughterhouses had glass walls, everyone would be a vegetarian.

> *Slaughterhouses in the United States produce an average of 3,700 calories per day for every man, woman, and child. The recommended daily allowance is 2,500 calories for men and 1,800 calories for women.*

People ask me all of the time whether I eat chicken. When I first started this program, I didn't intend to give up chicken. But about two and a half years after I gave up red meat, chicken started to taste funny to me. Its texture made it seem way too hard to digest, and the smell and taste just didn't appeal to me anymore, so I gave it up. At that time there were very few "free-range" chicken products available. Today, I still don't eat chicken, and I don't really recommend it in the long run for women because it is too concentrated a protein for females. My husband and sons eat a little of chicken every week as long as it is free-range. It's important that the chicken is free-range because not only are the chickens raised on natural grains and allowed to run free (hence, free-range), but they are killed in a humane and sanitary way.

> According to the U.S. Department of Agriculture, more than 8 billion animals are killed by the animal agriculture industry in the United States every year.

Have you ever wondered how a non-free-range chicken is killed? The natural life span of a chicken is thirteen to fifteen years. Most chickens are slaughtered when they are six or seven weeks old! The birds are crowded with other birds in cages and shipped to a processing plant. When they arrive at the plant, they often have the feces of those other birds on their feathers and skin. Then the birds are hung by their feet and stunned, so that they become brain dead, although they are very much alive.

After their blood is drained, the carcasses enter huge tanks where they are scalded. All the contamination on the bird's carcass goes right into that tank with each and every bird. (Think of it as fecal soup!) Although the water is hot enough to loosen their feathers, it is often not hot enough to kill all the bacteria. The scalding process opens feather follicles to aid feather removal, but also allows microorganisms to seep in and remain in the bird. The defeathering process is usually done mechanically, with machines that use little rubber fingers to pluck the chickens. Those fingers are not cleaned very often, and they collect bacteria like a magnet. They pass bacteria on to birds through their pores, crevices, and folds of skin.

Machines also remove the intestinal tract and organs. Washing is done at various stages of the process to try to remove contamination, but it is really more of a surface cleansing. Finally, the birds are chilled in large vats of water called immersion chillers. Salmonella and campylobacter get distributed between the chilling carcasses. Chlorine is often used to minimize the cross-contamination, but there are questions regarding its effectiveness and the possible chemical residue it leaves.

Good Nonmeat Sources of Protein

Almost all foods, except pure sugar and pure fat, contain some protein. A protein deficiency is basically unheard of in this country. Animal proteins are high in saturated fat, which of course makes them a major contributing factor to heart disease in humans. The proteins in animal products are highly concentrated, and most people who eat meat take in far more protein than they need or can handle.

Plant proteins, however, are associated with dietary fiber and contribute one of the most important elements to a healthy diet. Nuts, grains, seeds, green leafy vegetables, tofu and other soy products, legumes, and potatoes are all good sources of protein, and can supply your body with easy-to-break-down plant protein that is easy to digest.

Adopting a meatless diet is no longer considered peculiar or even exceptional. The American Dietetic Association has long held that a carefully planned vegetarian diet can be healthful and nutritionally sound. In fact, in 1996, the government finally gave vegetarianism an official nod of approval, according to its revised dietary guidelines. There are three basic types of vegetarianism. Veganism, the strictest form, excludes all animal products, including dairy products. Lactovegetarianism excludes meat, fish, poultry, and eggs, but allows other dairy products. A lacto-ovovegetarian diet excludes meat, fish, and poultry, but allows eggs and dairy. I consider myself a cross between a vegan vegetarian and one who follows most of the principles of macrobiotics, because I do not eat meat, chicken, dairy, or egg yolks, but I do eat fish and egg whites. This is what works for me.

People become vegetarians for a variety of reasons. A recent Gallup poll cited the main reason: It's good for your health. Many of the people polled also said they prefer the taste of vegetables to meat. A vegetarian diet can also reduce your blood cholesterol level, because a meatless diet is lower in fat and calories. It can keep cholesterol from doing any further harm, particularly the LDL cholesterol, which causes clogging of the arteries. Fruits and vegetables, staples of a vegetarian diet, contain numerous antioxidant nutrients, like beta-carotene, and vitamins C and E. Vegetarians usually have lower blood pressure than nonvegetarians do, partly because they tend to weigh less and perhaps because they consume less salt. (Their diet has become more balanced and they crave less of the extreme flavors of salt and meat.) But when meat eaters switch to a vegetarian diet, their blood pressure drops even if they don't lose weight or reduce their salt intake, apparently because plant foods are high in fiber, potassium, and magnesium, all of which are believed to lower blood pressure. Of course, a vegetarian diet also reduces your risk of cancer, diabetes, and coronary disease.

If you want to gradually start eating a vegetarian diet, make plant foods the center of your meal and cut back on the meat until you can easily just cut it out of your diet for good. If you do continue to eat meat, make sure you select lean cuts, and eat small portions. Cutting back on your meat intake could actually boost calcium levels. Animal protein tends to deplete calcium, so heavy meat eaters end up washing much of what they consume out of their system because it can't be absorbed. Vegetarians tend to have stronger, healthier bones.

8 STEP 5: The Miracle of Dairy-Free

*B*efore you start reading this chapter, if you are still a milk drinker, go pour yourself a big tall cold glass. Enjoy it, because I am absolutely certain that it will be your last. I have been virtually dairy-free since 1979, and believe me when I tell you unequivocally that eliminating dairy from your diet will change your life forever. It'll change the way you look, how you feel, and add years to your life. This is the chapter in my book where I am going to give you the down-and-dirty, in-your-face facts on why I believe dairy could kill. Think of this as the definitive "Anti-Milk Manifesto."

Almost every single person I talk to about this program invariably says to me, "There is no way I could ever give up milk or cheese." The overwhelming response from everyone is that they might be able to deal with all the other aspects of this health makeover, but the dairy thing, well, that just seems downright impossible! And I should know . . . When a nutritionist first suggested (based on my family history and what he could "read in my face") that I give up dairy, I was one of those people! But after reading about the connection between dairy and heart disease and dairy and arthritis, I decided, "What the hell . . . I'll try it for three months."

I used to love cheese, especially Jarlsberg and Brie. In fact, I loved dairy so much that I used to buy "cheese ends" at my local gourmet food shop. So, less than three months after giving it up (I couldn't even go the distance, that's how addicted to dairy I was!), I decided I just had to have a night of unabashed Jarlsberg. I ate three big bites of it, and I thought, "Oh my God! This is like eating my shoe!" It just tasted disgusting to me. The smell was funny (like feet) and the consistency was weird. I remember lying in bed that night, writhing with stomach pain. I made a deal with God that if He'd just let me digest this sludge, I promised never to eat dairy again! (I didn't have dairy after that until I went to Europe in 1982. After two or three days of eating cheese, I said, "This just isn't me anymore. Who do I think I am just because I'm in Europe to be eating like this?") Once I finally got off dairy for good, my face changed so much. That baby fat layer brought on and carried because of dairy consumption went away. I had bone structure that I never had before. My lungs and kidneys were functioning better because they got unclogged from that dairy sludge that was blocking their function.

Everyone who goes off dairy talks to me about having more energy, having better digestion, and feeling less stuffy in the nose. I can't think of anyone who didn't feel a difference. People might not stay completely dairy-free, but they never go back to where they were in the amount of dairy they used to eat. They know in the back of their heads that they shouldn't be eating dairy, and I'm certain that with each bite, there's a little voice saying, "Don't tell Marilu!"

I was at Fran Drescher's home for dinner one night (she's a fabulous cook and absolutely gorgeous without one stitch of makeup), and she had put some cheese in the salad. Fran asked me why I didn't want any of the cheese. I went into my usual spiel on dairy (P.S. I've ruined many dinner parties with this speech!), which goes a little something like this.

The only thing milk is supposed to do is to turn a 50-pound calf into a 300-pound cow in six months. If cows don't drink milk, why would you? If I offered you a cold glass of breast milk, would you drink it? Okay, maybe you might, but what if I offered you dog's milk or orangutan's milk? (Frankly, it makes more sense that we would drink orangutan's milk because we are closer to them as a species than we are to a cow.) Humans were never meant to consume anything other than human breast milk, and only while we're babies. We are the only animals on earth that drink the milk of another animal (except for the domesticated cat and they shouldn't drink it either). Milk is a food of convenience, and in our quest for convenience, we have made ourselves one of the sickest animals on the face of the earth. In many countries (like India and China), the thought of drinking milk from a cow is as absurd as drinking milk from an orangutan.

> *Milk is nature's food for a baby calf, which has four stomachs, and will double its weight in forty-seven days.*

Not only does a baby calf have four stomachs, it also has nine feet of intestines, as opposed to humans, who have twenty-seven feet of intestines. Our digestive enzymes are not capable of breaking down a food that is designed to nurse the young of another species. Our stomachs don't even recognize dairy as a "food," and everything we eat with it has a difficult time being digested.

The fat and cholesterol contained in milk is a real one-two punch to the human body. Genetically speaking, milk is identical to the human growth hormone IGF-I. Sixty percent of America's dairy cows have the leukemia virus. Their bodies are grossly injected with steroids and antibiotics, which they pass on in their milk. Pasteurization is intended to kill bacteria and viruses in milk, but in recent years we have heard countless stories of contaminated beef and diseases attributed to eating beef or drinking tainted dairy products. Here are some startling statistics that might grab your attention. By the time the average American reaches the age of fifty-two, he or she has consumed, in milk and dairy products, the equivalent cholesterol contained in 1 million slices of bacon. Twenty-five million American women over the age of forty have been diagnosed with bone-crippling arthritis and osteo-porosis. On the average, these women consumed two pounds of milk per day their entire adult lives.

Many dairy cows graze on pesticide-infested grass and drink contaminated water. These cows become so contaminated that their milk can be a near-lethal brew. Milk is loaded with pus from cows that have mastitis (ulcers on cow's udders), which is then treated with antibiotics. It contains bacteria, and despite the numerous wonder drugs that cows are treated with, the bacteria is not entirely destroyed.

By now you must be thinking to yourself, "What about all the good things we hear about milk, like it helps build calcium and keeps our bones strong?" Although millions of dollars are spent every year trumpeting the virtues of milk, the truth is that the cal-cium in cow's milk is much coarser than calcium in human milk, and the human body does not adequately absorb it. Also, all the processing of dairy products reduces the calcium supply in those products, so it becomes very difficult to use pasteurized, homoge-nized, or other processed dairy products as a good source of cal-cium. In fact, most of us could get enough calcium through other foods we eat, so we don't need to get it from milk. Spinach, broc-coli, and all other green leafy vegetables contain calcium. Nuts and sesame seeds are also great sources of calcium. Even concentrated fruits like dates, figs, and prunes offer enough calcium for your body's needs. Cows get *their* calcium from eating grass in the fields where they graze, so we are actually getting it once removed. (You don't really think they're getting their calcium from eating a Christmas cheese log, do you?) Next time you go to drink a glass of milk, think of it as orangutan milk or doggie milk. Wake up, America, because it's time to wipe off your milk mustache . . . for good.

What's the Matter with Milk?

Milk, in all its glory, has become synonymous with America, Mom, and apple pie. Too bad for us, because milk could actually be the cause of many ailments we suffer from as adults (and as children). The consumption of milk and dairy products has been linked to a variety of problems. Dairy products can cause respiratory problems, canker sores, skin conditions, and other allergic reactions. And those are the small afflictions associated with dairy. Heart disease, arthritis, childhood diabetes, kidney stones, allergies, depression and mood swings, and, worst of all, Jacob-Cruetzfeldt disease (mad cow disease) have all been seriously linked to milk and dairy. Breast cancer, insulin-dependent diabetes, ovarian cancer, and even osteoporosis have also been linked to dairy consumption.

At least 50 percent of all children in the United States are allergic to milk, and many go undiagnosed until it's too late. One out of every five babies suffers from colic, and cow's milk is often the reason. Eliminating cow's milk formulas will solve the problem, but taking the *baby* off milk isn't the only answer. If a breast-feeding mother drinks a lot of milk, she can pass the cows' antibodies through her breast milk on to the nursing child. The mother needs to stop drinking milk, too. (I always found it ridiculous to tell pregnant and nursing mothers to drink a lot of milk. Cows eat grass to make their milk. You don't have to *drink* milk to *make* milk!) Dairy products are the leading cause of food allergies in this country. Such allergies can bring on diarrhea, constipation, and chronic fatigue. Asthma and sinus infections are also associated with dairy, because it becomes mucus-forming in the human body. (I get a kick out of people telling me that they're not allergic to dairy, and ten minutes after chomping on a slice of pizza, or sucking down a "grande latte," they start sneezing.) Some people actually force themselves to drink milk because they still really believe it's good for them.

According to recent studies, about one in three cartons of milk available at your local grocery store contains some of the antibiotics that were fed to the cows back on the farm. Dairies add vitamin D to milk, and if they add too much, it can be potentially fatal. A sip of milk contains hundreds of different substances. Separately, each one has the potential to have a biological effect on us. Together, all these proteins and hormones and fat, cholesterol, viruses, bacteria, pesticides, and added vitamin D combine to affect us in ways far beyond our own comprehension. Pasteurizing milk destroys the vitamins in it. That's why we have to artificially add back the vitamin D. But a startling number of dairies are not adding the right amount of vitamin D. A recent Boston University Medical School study showed that 71 percent of milk samples tested from five eastern states dairies contained significantly too much vitamin D (61 percent) or too little (10 percent). A subsequent study of those same dairies run months later showed that 25 percent of them were still not getting it right. Excess vitamin D is stored in body fat, so it can take months or even years to clear out the toxic surplus. Vitamin D is important because it regulates the absorption of dietary calcium in our bodies. Without it, efforts to eat enough calcium are useless, and too much vitamin D causes calcium to accumulate in the blood and urine and can eventually lead to kidney failure. That seems like a high price to pay for drinking a glass of milk!

CALCIUM IN FOODS

Vegetables	Calcium (mg)
Broccoli (1 cup, boiled)	178
Brussels sprouts (8 sprouts)	56
Carrots (2 medium)	38
Cauliflower (1 cup, boiled)	34
Celery (1 cup, boiled)	54
Collards (1 cup, boiled)	148
Kale (1 cup, boiled)	94
Onions (1 cup, boiled)	58

Vegetables	Calcium (mg)
Potato, baked (1 medium)	20
Romaine lettuce (1 cup)	20
Squash, butternut (1 cup, boiled)	84
Sweet potato (1 cup, boiled)	70

Legumes	
Chickpeas (1 cup, canned)	78
Great northern beans (1 cup, boiled)	121
Green beans (1 cup, boiled)	58
Kidney beans (1 cup, boiled)	50
Lentils (1 cup, boiled)	37
Lima beans (1 cup, boiled)	52
Navy beans (1 cup, boiled)	128
Peas, green (1 cup, boiled)	44
Pinto beans (1 cup, boiled)	82
Soybeans (1 cup, boiled)	175
Turtle beans, black (1 cup, boiled)	103
Tofu ($\frac{1}{2}$ cup)	258
Vegetarian baked beans (1 cup)	128
Wax beans (1 cup, canned)	174
White beans (1 cup, boiled)	161

Grains	
Brown rice (cooked, 1 cup)	23
Corn bread (1 2-ounce piece)	133
Corn tortilla (1 medium)	42
English muffin (1 medium)	92
Pancake mix ($\frac{1}{4}$ cup, 3 pancakes)	140
Pita bread (1 piece)	31
Wheat bread (1 slice)	30
Wheat flour, all-purpose (1 cup)	22
Wheat flour, calcium-enriched (1 cup)	238
Whole-wheat flour (1 cup)	49

Fruits	Calcium (mg)
Apple (1 medium)	10
Banana (1 medium)	7
Figs, dried (10 medium)	269
Orange, navel (1 medium)	56
Orange juice, calcium-fortified (1 cup)	300
Pear (1 medium)	19
Raisins (2/3 cup)	53

CALCIUM MAY BE BENEFICIAL FOR THE FOLLOWING AILMENTS

Body Part/System	Ailment
Blood/circulatory system	Anemia
	Diabetes
	Hemophilia
	Pernicious anemia
Bones	Backache
	Fracture
	Osteomalacia
	Osteoporosis
Bowel	Colitis
	Diarrhea
Brain/nervous system	Dizziness
	Epilepsy
	Finger tremors
	Insomnia
	Irritability
	Mental illness
	Nervousness
	Parkinson's disease
Ear	Meniere's syndrome
Eye	Cataracts
Head	Headache

Body Part/System	Ailment
Heart	Arteriosclerosis
	Atherosclerosis
	Hypertension
	LDL levels, high
Intestine	Cancer (large intestine)
	Celiac disease
	Constipation
	Hemorrhoids
	Worms
Joints	Arthritis
	Rheumatism
Kidney	Nephritis
Leg	Growing pains
	Leg cramps
Lungs/respiratory system	Allergies
	Common cold
	Tuberculosis
Muscles	General muscle cramps
	Tetany
Nails	Nail problems
Skin	Acne
	Bee and spider bites
	Sunburn
Stomach	Stomach ulcer (peptic)
Teeth/gums	Brittle teeth
	Cavities
	Pyorrhea
	Tooth and gum disorders
General	Aging
	Fever
	Overweight and obesity
	Toxicity

So what exactly is in a glass of milk? The following chart shows the average daily intake of various components found in milk. The average American eats approximately 2.5 pounds of dairy and dairy-based products every day.

WHAT'S IN A GLASS OF MILK?

Ingredient	Amount Per Serving	Daily Average of Milk Products
Water	87.2%	N/A
Calories	66	749.10
Protein	3.5 grams	39.73 grams
Fat	3.7 grams	42 grams
Carbohydrate	4.9 grams	55.62 grams
Calcium	117 mg	1,327.95 mg
Phosphorus	92 mg	1,044.20 mg
Iron	Trace	Trace
Sodium	50 mg	567.50 mg
Potassium	140 mg	1,589 mg
Vitamin A	150.01 IU	1,702.50 IU
Thiamin	.03 mg	.34 mg
Riboflavin	.17 mg	1.93 mg
Niacin	.10 mg	1.14 mg
Ascorbic acid	1 mg	11.35 mg

Based on 100 grams (3.3 oz) of whole milk.

Milk has been referred to as liquid meat. It contains the same amino acids and protein as meat. It's no wonder, since it comes from the same place. Besides the ingredients listed in the chart above, milk also contains a surplus of hormones. Each sip of milk has pituitary, hypothalamic, pancreatic, thyroid, parathyroid, adrenal, gonadal, and gut hormones in it. Besides these hormones, cow's milk contains a variety of proteins and protein hormones, including steroid hormones like progesterone, calcitonin, and estrogen.

Bovine Slime

Of course, many of you may have also heard something about the bovine growth hormones that are injected into cows. (If you drink milk, you won't grow an extra limb or another head, but these hormones are not good for you!) They can cause premature growth in children and abnormal proliferation of intestinal cells. Milk has virtually become genetically engineered. These hormones are given to the cows to make them get fat and produce up to 20 percent more milk. The human body has its own agenda for proper growth. It doesn't need extra hormones sending it messages. Approximately 25 percent of dairy cows use Posilac (the trade name for rBGH, the dangerous growth hormone) to boost milk production. The first company to manufacture Posilac, Monsanto, will earn in excess of $500 million annually from this one product in the United States *alone*. Considering the fact that we make too much milk already, why are we injecting hormones that are unhealthy to increase production of milk? In the mid-1800s, the average cow yielded just under *two quarts* of milk per day. By 1960, the yield was just over *nine quarts* per day. Today, cows can yield up to *fifty quarts* of milk a day. That's an average of 18,000 pounds of milk per cow, per year. It's forced, it's unnatural, and it's definitely unhealthy! (Guess you're not having a *milk* shake with that *burger* you're not eating, huh, Oprah?)

> *Dr. Benjamin Spock, well-known pediatrician, has publicly announced that, in his opinion, "an infant should not be fed cow's milk during the first year of life."*

By the way, from whom do you think the dairy farmers get the money when they sell their surplus of 9 billion pounds of milk each year? You, that's who. The government uses your tax dollars to pay the dairy farmers. In addition to buying the surplus, the government also spends $1.3 billion every year to slaughter 1 million diseased or dysfunctional cows that were producing the surplus. You know what happens to them? They get ground up and processed and are fed back to other cows! This is really an important issue, because cows are vegetarians; they are not carnivores. The farmer has turned them against their nature by feeding them beef. (That's *CANNIBALISM!*) Aside from that, the cows are eating the meat of diseased animals. They are milked and pass on the disease in the process. Intellectually, drinking milk just doesn't make sense.

Dairy and the Cancer Connection

Dairy food may be one of the most potent factors in the development of breast cancer. A study of 250 women in Vercelli, Italy, with breast cancer found that they tended to consume considerably more milk, high-fat cheese, and butter than 499 healthy women from the same region of Italy. Breast cancer risks tripled among women who consumed about half their calories in fat, 13–23 percent of their calories as saturated fat, and 8–20 percent of their calories as animal protein. On the contrary, a diet high in complex carbohydrates and soybeans *reduced* the incidence of breast cancer in laboratory experiments. British researchers reported that the natural phytoestrogens found in whole grains and soybean products, such as tofu, can have a major effect on hormonal activity, and are believed to be a great tool in fighting the war on cancer. Researchers at Harvard have found that women who consume large amounts of cottage cheese and yogurt increase their risk of ovarian cancer by up to three times. Ovarian cancer is strongly correlated with lactase persistence and per capita milk consumption, which, simply put, points the finger at dairy products rather than fat as the key dietary variable for developing ovarian cancer. (In other words, you still run a risk if you drink even 1 percent or skim milk.)

Another link to cancer might come from the fact that dairy farmers use so many hormones to pump up their cows in order to make more milk. These hormones that we're ingesting stimulate growth hormones in our body that can mutate and cause deformed cellular growth and cancerous tumors to develop.

Dairy and Nutrient Deficiencies

Someone who eats a dairy-rich diet is more likely to develop an iron deficiency. Cow's milk products are very low in iron. It contains only 0.10 milligram per eight-ounce serving. The U.S. Recommended Daily Allowance is fifteen milligrams. An infant would have to drink thirty-one quarts of milk a day to get the recommended daily amount of iron. But the iron deficiency caused by milk isn't just because of its low iron content. Milk has a tendency to displace iron-rich foods. Milk could also cause a loss of blood from the intestinal tract, which can reduce the amount of iron the body stores over time. Researchers think that the blood loss may be caused by bovine albumin, a protein present in milk, which may elicit an immune reaction that can lead to blood loss. Milk and cheese will reduce the amount of iron absorbed by the body by approximately half.

Breast Feeding and Dairy

One of the greatest experiences I've had as a mother was being able to breast feed both of my sons until they were almost a year old. The love, the bonding, and the connection a mother feels to her child is made that much richer when she knows that she is giving her child the greatest gift of all, his or her future health. I am very pro breast feeding. Not only did I dedicate an entire show to the subject when I had my own talk show, but I received an award from La Leche League. (This is an incredible national organization that helps women learn how to breast feed and take care of themselves during this time as well.) Mother's milk is a perfect food to nurture an infant. If you must use a formula, there are many that are not dairy-based. Substituting cow's milk for mother's breast milk is a key factor in the abnormally increasing body size of humans, both in weight and in height. The size of certain cells in the body is determined by the foods we eat early in life, and eating food that contains unnatural and unhealthy growth hormones surely is a factor in developing oversized cells. An excessive amount of these cells can lead to an obese and unhealthy teenager as well as an overweight adult. Children who drank cow's milk are consistently more overweight than children who were breast fed as infants. Once you wean your child from breast feeding, it isn't an invitation to introduce him to dairy.

Milk and dairy products are the leading cause of allergies in children. Dairy foods sensitize the mucus membranes in a child and increase their sensitivity to other foreign substances, like pollen or dust. You might notice that kids who eat a lot of dairy growing up are more prone to ear infections, colds, or other respiratory infections.

Breast feeding greatly reduces the risk of certain cancers for both mother and child. Researchers from the National Institute of Child Health and Human Development in Bethesda, Maryland, have found that infants breast fed more than six months had a lower risk of developing cancer in childhood, especially lymphomas. In this study, children who were formula fed, or breast fed less than six months, had approximately twice the risk of getting some childhood cancers by age fifteen as those who were breast fed for longer than six months. They also have five times the risk of getting lymphoma. Mother's milk contains substantial antimicrobial benefits for infants, increasing their resistance to many infections and possibly protecting them from many diseases. A Chinese medical study found that the longer a mother nurses, the less at risk she was for developing breast cancer.

Fat and Dairy Products

The fat found in dairy products is animal fat, which is high in cholesterol. Whole milk and anything made from whole milk is very high in saturated fat, which can increase your cholesterol level. "Saturated" is a chemical term that means the fat molecule is completely covered with hydrogen atoms. Without those atoms, the fat is "unsaturated." Saturated fats stimulate your liver to make more cholesterol. Most animal products contain substantial amounts of saturated fat. Lose dairy, and you'll lose fat. (For more information about fat, see Chapter 10 on fat.)

Making butter requires 21.2 pounds of milk for each "finished" pound of butter. One quart of milk weighs 2.15 pounds.

So, the end of my Fran Drescher story is that she said, "I'm going to try that [eliminating dairy products]." A few weeks later she called and said, "I feel such a difference, I can't believe it!" She was so convinced she wrote about it in her book too!

All I can say is God bless Weight Watchers, Marilyn, "my therapist," and Marilu Henner for contributing to the changes in my thinking about food. Over a dinner at our house, Marilu began to tell us about her miracle diet. I had to comment on how great she looked so soon after giving birth. But there, Marilu sat chattering away in tight, black jeans, a ball of energy with a clear and beautiful complexion, and proceeded to tell us that she had eliminated all dairy from her diet. Marilu said, "If you want to see the weight drop off, have boundless energy, a faster metabolic rate, and reduce significantly any allergies you might be suffering from, you'll try it, and within six months, you won't believe the changes." My only response to her was "not even Parmesan on pasta?" "You can get a substitute made of soy," she answered with a straight face. We started right after a trip to Martha's Vineyard and I've been happily dairy-free ever since. P.S. It's everything she claimed it would be, and then some. My skin got thinner, my face got clearer, and much to my relief, I don't crave cheese.

FRAN DRESCHER,
EXCERPT FROM HER BOOK
ENTER WHINING (REGANBOOKS)

And for those of you who think you can't give up dairy, the changes that you will see in your body, your face, your energy level, and your total health ought to be the greatest incentive. Plus, I believe that dairy is the most effective first step if you're going to try only one of my steps. (Dairy and food combining are the dynamic duo.) It's pretty easy to experiment with giving up dairy, because it's something you can cut back on until you finally do away with dairy products all together. Try dipping your bread in a little olive oil instead of butter. Order a "cheeseless" pizza (they're not as hard to find as you might think, and they're delicious! Even Domino's will make one for you!). Make your kids a grilled soy cheese sandwich. I'll bet they'll eat it and enjoy it, too! For those of you still drinking coffee (I hope you've at least switched to decaf), who need a little milk, try Rice Dream or soy milk. (They even offer it at Starbucks.) Your body will thank you! As the ad says, "Got Milk?" *No thanks!*

❋　❋　❋　❋　❋　❋　❋　❋　❋　❋

HOW DAIRY-FREE LIVING CHANGED MY LIFE

Real people comment on their experience of giving up dairy (if it worked for them, it will work for you!).

The first thing I stopped was dairy for two weeks. I thought, "What's the worst thing that can happen?" At first it was kind of confusing, because I was eating more grains. For everything you love, there's a substitute. I never feel

deprived. But it became like an addiction for me, because once I got that increase in my energy and saw the results, I knew I would never go back to eating dairy!

MAGGIE GILLOTT FOUNTAIN,
age forty-two, registered nurse,
who lost fifty-five pounds

I rarely eat dairy and have been this way since the early 1980s. I even followed this lifestyle during my pregnancies. If I eat dairy now and I have the slightest hint of a cold, I find that it only exacerbates it. I notice a big positive difference in my skin when I'm staying dairy-free.

CHRISTAL WELLAND,
director, Merrill Lynch

I like to refer to this program as living "mucus-free." Stopping dairy was a big thing for me. I saw such quick results when I stopped eating dairy products. I had so much energy, and that's what made me stick with it. The first thing that people noticed was my face. I got my face back. I lost my double chin, and my stomach is more refined. I look healthier and feel great!

JIM BORSTELMANN,
professional dancer and cast member
of the Broadway musical *Chicago*

Cheese was really hard for me to give up. I like the taste, texture, and feel of it in my mouth. What dairy does to your internal organs is an incredible deterrent. Knowing how bad dairy is for me made it easier for me to make the choice to abstain. I'm enjoying soy cheese and other nondairy products more than I thought I would.

LILLIE KAE STEVENS,
professional actress, singer, dancer, and
cast member of the Broadway musical *Chicago*

When I saw how Marilu changed, it got my attention. Dairy was one of the last holdouts for me. I slowly cut it out from my diet. I was down to just eating frozen yogurt and putting a little milk in my coffee. When I saw the results from cutting back, I knew I had to go all the way. I gave up caffeine, which forced me to give up milk in my coffee (since I wasn't drinking it anymore). Eating out isn't a problem, either. You simply order your food and ask for no dairy. I love the way I feel about myself, and I'm raising my kids without dairy. They're healthy, vibrant kids!

MARY ANN HENNINGS,
professional hairstylist for television
and film, who lost twenty pounds

❊　　❊　　❊　　❊　　❊　　❊　　❊　　❊　　❊　　❊

Dairy Alternatives

So now that I've got you thinking about getting off milk, does this mean your days of ice cream, cheese pizza, and cappuccinos are over? Good news . . . you can have all of the above. There are many dairy substitutes on the market today. Soy, rice, oats, and almonds are all used to make dairy substitute products. Giving up dairy only means you're giving up "traditional" dairy that comes from a cow or other animals. A mecca of products is readily available, and they are really very good tasting, too.

Milk

Milk as a beverage can be replaced by soy milk, which comes plain or flavored. Rice milk (especially Rice Dream Original Flavor) is also a good substitute. Vita-Soy and Eden Soy are good low-fat soy milks. Companies such as Imagine Foods make easy-to-drink packages that look like juice boxes.

Cheese

Louis Lanza, owner of Josie's restaurant in New York City, (and a contributor to this book—see the selection of recipes from Josie's in Appendix B), specializes in creating nondairy meals. He catered a party for me between the two shows we do on Wednesdays for the cast and crew of *Chicago*. Everyone walked in and saw these incredible-looking dishes, some of them draped in cheese. If I hadn't told everyone that they were eating soy cheese, they would never have known.

Another substitute for cheese can be a variety of dips and spreads such as hummus (made from chickpeas) or tahini (a spread made from sesame). You can also use peas, lentils, avocado, or other kinds of beans for spreads and dips.

Eggs

True vegetarians consider eggs dairy. Others do not. You can decide for yourself if you want to eat eggs. I occasionally have an egg-white omelet for breakfast. It's up to you on this one. Eggs can easily be eliminated from your diet. Tofu has about the same consistency and can have many different flavors depending on what you eat with it. Foods such as pancakes and cakes can easily be made without using eggs. If you're looking to use eggs as a binding agent while cooking, try using egg whites only, or substituting with potato starch, cornstarch, or kuzu. Oat or wheat flour can also be used, as can mashed potatoes and even tapioca pudding, depending on the recipe. For baking, lightness can be achieved by using extra yeast or baking soda. Fruit juice can also be used to replace any liquid needs from milk. Eggs can be simulated by replacing their need in a recipe with any of the following formulas (equal to one egg):

* One teaspoon arrowroot powder, one teaspoon soy powder, and one-quarter cup water.

* One-quarter cup soaked soy beans or garbanzo beans blended with one-quarter cup water.

* One tablespoon tahini and three tablespoons of any liquid (such as juice).

* Two ounces tofu blended with any liquid.

* One-half banana, mashed.

Butter

The easiest and best substitute for butter is vegetable oil, especially olive, safflower, and canola oils. There are also vegetable-oil soy margarines like Shedd's Willow Run or Hain Margarine.

Mayonnaise

Tofu or cooked potatoes are the most common replacements for mayo. Nayonnaise is an easy-to-find substitute, and the best tasting.

Ice Cream

I swear to you that soy ice cream tastes better than most frozen yogurt! If you try it, you'll become an instant convert. There are some really good brands available, like the Imagine foods version called Rice Dream. (They even have a line of puddings available that will knock you out.) If you have a taste for a milk shake, try a fruit smoothie using fresh fruit and Rice Dream. You can add some nuts if you want, for extra flavor.

❋　❋　❋　❋　❋　❋　❋　❋　❋　❋

GLOSSARY OF SOME INGREDIENTS
USED IN THE SUBSTITUTES

Tofu
A soybean cheese. It's similar to cottage cheese in its consistency, preparation, and taste.

Tahini
A sesame butter that can be spread like regular butter or mixed with other ingredients to make spreads, sauces, or protein drinks.

Miso
A salty soybean paste that can be used to make spreads, sauces, and soups.

❋　❋　❋　❋　❋　❋　❋　❋　❋　❋

I can't promise you that you'll be crazy about every dairy substitute I talked about here, but you might be surprised at how good they taste once you give them a try. Soy ice cream is not your favorite flavor of Häagen-Dazs, but it isn't a bad substitute, and given the health hazards of eating dairy, I'd hardly say real ice cream is worth the risk. It'll take a little experimenting and tasting to find the substitutes you like and don't like.

9 | STEP 6: Food Combining— The Winning Combination

9 first learned about food combining from a book called *Ten Talents* that my sister's boyfriend gave me for Christmas 1979. (He was the only true vegetarian I knew at the time.) *Ten Talents* was written in the 1930s and contained a simple, natural approach to food that the world seems to be embracing (and trying to get back to) today. This book outlined everything I needed to know about the value of eating food that is properly combined.

The basic idea is to think of each meal as either a fruit, a starch, or a protein meal. It was an unusual way to approach eating, because it was the exact opposite of the typical American diet. I grew up in the Midwest eating meat and potatoes, spaghetti and meatballs, and turkey sandwiches. Any other "diet" I ever read about always included a protein exchange, a bread exchange, and fruit exchange for dessert. (I'll explain later why most diets purposely do this.) *Ten Talents* explained that food combining not only was the healthiest way to eat, but that I would lose weight and have more energy (or "Hennergy," as my family likes to call it) in the process. This wasn't a diet about counting calories or about portion control. It was about respecting the chemical properties of each food and how each food reacts when combined with other foods. When I let my mind wander and made up meals in my head that stayed within the rules, it was hard to believe that it could actually work. I told my girlfriend Barbara about what I had read, and with her as a willing partner-in-crime, I put this theory to the test, and tried really extreme versions of food combinations. We'd have an all-starch night at our favorite Italian restaurant that included potatoes, pasta, vodka, and bread. We tried an all-fish night when we ate smoked salmon as an appetizer, grilled swordfish for dinner, and a salad with tuna sashimi for dessert. To my shock and total amazement . . . it worked! I knew that this was an eating program I could live with the rest of my life. This was *a lifestyle change*, not just another fad diet.

Why Food Combining?

After trying food combining for a while, I felt lighter and more balanced, and I wanted to feel that way forever. I felt stronger, I stood up straighter, and I really felt better about myself, and, believe me, it showed in *everything* I did. The amount of weight that I lost was incredible, and the weight loss came naturally with all the other benefits. If you perfectly food combine, you won't believe the results. Your digestion will work so much better (remember, something goes in, something gets processed, something comes out) and the volume of food you can eat will surprise you. You lose that gassy, bloated, stomach-distended feeling. Suddenly, your food starts working for you, not against you.

If you think I am completely out of my mind, let me say that food combining theories date back to the early 1800s. Those were times when there was little, if any, understanding of food digestion and assimilation. The name may have changed over the years, but food combining is a concept that has survived through every fad diet that has come and gone. With all the information about nutrition that constantly bombards us, there are no excuses for not eating a healthy, well-balanced, centered diet. (Anyone who is still defending his or her right to eat an unhealthy diet is the one who's *crazy!*) Everything you will read and hear about food combining makes it sound so logical, it will seem incomprehensible that you don't already live your life that way. The principles of a proper food combining diet are easy to follow once you have a grasp of the basics. The best thing is that you get to eat more food than when you are on a "typical" diet, but you'll also be eating less food than when you pig out. It allows you to eat more volume on a daily basis, but not in that feast-or-famine, crazy out-of-control way, unless one night you have to . . . then see Chapter 13 on gusto.

How Food Combining Works

The theory behind food combining was popularized by Dr. William Hay in the 1920s. He suffered from high blood pressure and heart problems, and through his experimentation with food combining, Dr. Hay discovered that within a matter of a few months, his weight had dropped significantly and his health had improved a great deal. Dr. Hay discovered that when protein and starches are eaten together, it takes too much energy to digest that meal. The body gets confused and cannot manufacture the necessary enzymes at the same time to properly digest the food. His findings showed that the undigested food just sat in the stomach for hours, rotting and unable to digest properly, which creates toxins in the bloodstream. Some digestion *does* take place, but partially through bacterial action, which causes fermentation that then causes such side effects as gas, bloating, and abdominal pain.

Bacterial digestion creates another important side effect— poisonous by-products, such as ptomaine and leucomaine. Bacterial fermentation of starch can also result in toxic by-products like acetic acid, lactic acid, and carbon dioxide. Proper food combining helps the body digest enzymatically, which produces essential amino acids that repair and maintain the body.

So what did all of this mean to Dr. Hay? (And ultimately to us?) The basic result behind Dr. Hay's research was that meat and potatoes were no longer feasible. A hamburger and french fries were a thing of his past. No more turkey and stuffing for Dr. Hay. He would be eating noodles with mushrooms, rice and vegetables, and meat with tomatoes. Years later, Dr. Herbert M. Shelton wrote *Food Combining Made Easy*, which became the basis of modern-day food combining theories. *Fit for Life* by Harvey and Marilyn Diamond sold millions of copies in the late 1980s, and brought the ideas of food combining into the mainstream.

Proper food combining (or eating the right foods together) ultimately enhances the nutritional value of well-digested food. Remember in Chapter 2, the "Balance" chapter, we talked about how important it is to have your "sanitation system" working, whether it's your apartment, your desk at work, or your body? Well, the only way to keep your body's sanitation system working properly is to understand that there are certain limitations to the efficiency of our digestive enzymes. We must learn to respect those limitations, eat accordingly, and help the body along in the process. When we eat the *wrong* foods together, the result is digestive trouble. We're so used to feeling lousy after a meal (stuffed, bloated, and gassy) that unless we feel that way, we don't feel we've eaten!

Eating certain foods together interferes with digestion, which ultimately leads to poor health and unwanted excess pounds. Eating "starch-rich" foods in combination with "protein-rich" foods is the most common mistake people make in their diet. Avoiding this mistake is the underlying premise behind food combining, because eating proteins and starches together unnecessarily taxes the digestive system. Proteins and starches require different digestive enzymes, which function at different pH levels in the body. Pepsin digests protein in the highly acidic environment of the stomach, and starches prefer alkaline environments such as the intestines. Combining these two types of food traps them and slows down the digestive process. The undigested food causes digestive problems such as gas, bloating, constipation, and weight gain. (That drama again!)

The digestive process zaps more energy from us than any other bodily function. Food combining is a simple plan to follow, and if practiced properly, will result in preserving your health and vitality. We don't need a lot of food to feel satiated (especially if the food we're eating is truly feeding us!). Food combining does not limit your choices in terms of what to eat, but only in what to eat together for the best results. I really believe that food combining is the healthiest approach to eating you can take. It's not a diet in the traditional sense because it allows you to eat a healthier amount of food than most other programs. Food combining gives you the best chance to digest everything you eat in a sensible, efficient, healthy way. It's a whole new way of approaching eating and food, which puts us closer to being "the animal we were meant to be."

My food combining program is designed to offer you the most effective method for digestive excellence. It is based on the same principles and eating patterns that our earliest ancestors lived by. This practice of eating a food alone or combined with only one or two other types of foods has been practiced for tens of thousands of years, and is the basis of our digestive capacities. As we've talked about so many times, we have gotten away from the way we're supposed to live. (Not that I'm saying, "Let's go back to the caveman days!") Our diet, our level of activity, the way we stand, walk, and so on, all fall short of the vibrant health that we're capable of achieving. This simple approach to eating is a return to the basics and the way our bodies were meant to eat and digest.

One really simple way to understand why food combining works is a lesson in Chemistry 101. Imagine your stomach as a beaker. When you eat a protein (fish, chicken, meat, eggs, dairy), your mouth sends a signal to the brain to put an acid base in the stomach to digest the protein. When you eat a starch (bread, potatoes, rice, pasta, grains), your mouth sends a different signal to the brain to send an alkaline base to digest it. *ACIDS AND ALKALINES NEUTRALIZE EACH OTHER!* When you eat proteins and starches together, everything gets neutralized and nothing gets digested. It's scientific.

We derive absolutely no nutritional value from undigested food. In fact, food that is left undigested just rots in our stomachs. (Yuck!) The rotting causes a toxic response by turning into poison and alcohol, leaving us with a toxic mess worse than Chernobyl to clean up. Once we eat, food has two choices: It either digests or it doesn't. Proper food combining leaves you with only one choice, and that is proper digestion. It also sets a stage for more energy and less weight. You will realize how wonderful food combining feels firsthand once you try it. I have seen it work on friends, family, and myself! Of my ten steps, if you try only food combining and eliminating dairy from your diet, you will not believe how dramatically your body will respond. Everyone who tries this program seems to agree that this one-two punch will get you closer to becoming that sleek, beautiful, healthy animal you were meant to be, and it is right at your doorstep (or on your plate).

> *I really believe in food combining. It's the most logical thing. If you eat ice cream with pickles and herring, and try to digest that, your body is going to digest that combination differently than if you ate any one of those separately. This is an extreme example, but it makes the point.*
>
> LORIN HENNER, MY BROTHER

> *Marilu turned me on to food combining, and whenever I want to lose weight fast and in a healthy way, I start on her food combining program and eliminate dairy from my diet. I can see results right away. Intellectually it just makes sense.*
>
> JOHN MATOIN, PRESIDENT OF HBO

The following are your best guidelines to food combining.

❋　❋　❋　❋　❋　❋　❋　❋　❋　❋

THE BASIC RULES OF FOOD COMBINING

1. Do *not* eat proteins and starches together. Your body requires an acid base to digest proteins and an alkaline base to digest starches. Proteins and starches combine well with green, leafy vegetables and nonstarchy vegetables, but they do not combine well with each other.

2. Do *not* mix fruit with proteins, starches, or any kind of vegetable. Fruits digest so quickly that by the time they reach your stomach, they are already partially digested. If they are combined with other foods, they will rot and ferment. *Only* eat fruit with other fruit.

3. Melons digest faster than any other food. Therefore, you should *never* eat melons with any other food, including other fruits. Always eat melons on their own.

4. Do *not* mix acid and/or sub-acid fruits with sweet fruits at the same meal. Acid fruits, such as grapefruits, pineapple, and strawberries, can be mixed with sub-acid fruits, such as apples, grapes, and peaches, but neither of these categories can be mixed with sweet fruits, such as bananas, dates, or raisins.

5. Eat only four to six different fruits or vegetables at one meal.

6. Fats and oils combine with everything (except fruits) but should be used in limited amounts because while they won't inhibit digestion, they will slow it down.

7. Wait the following lengths of time between meals that don't combine:
   a. Two hours after eating fruit.
   b. Three hours after eating starches.
   c. Four hours after eating proteins.

❋　❋　❋　❋　❋　❋　❋　❋　❋　❋

MARILU HENNER'S FOOD-COMBINING CHART

CHART 1

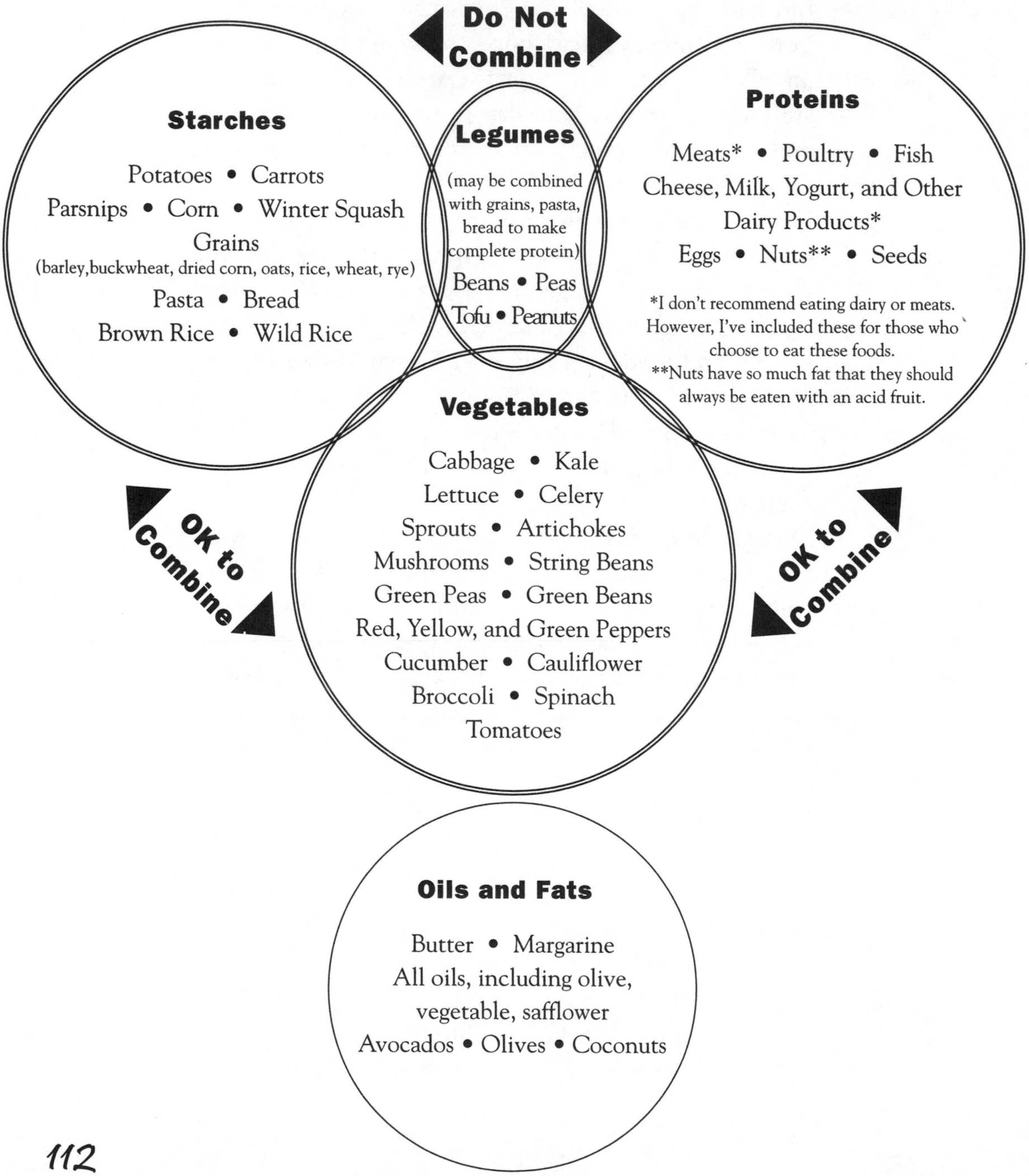

◄ **Do Not Combine** ►

Starches

Potatoes • Carrots
Parsnips • Corn • Winter Squash
Grains
(barley, buckwheat, dried corn, oats, rice, wheat, rye)
Pasta • Bread
Brown Rice • Wild Rice

Legumes

(may be combined with grains, pasta, bread to make complete protein)

Beans • Peas
Tofu • Peanuts

Proteins

Meats* • Poultry • Fish
Cheese, Milk, Yogurt, and Other
Dairy Products*
Eggs • Nuts** • Seeds

*I don't recommend eating dairy or meats.
However, I've included these for those who
choose to eat these foods.
**Nuts have so much fat that they should
always be eaten with an acid fruit.

Vegetables

Cabbage • Kale
Lettuce • Celery
Sprouts • Artichokes
Mushrooms • String Beans
Green Peas • Green Beans
Red, Yellow, and Green Peppers
Cucumber • Cauliflower
Broccoli • Spinach
Tomatoes

OK to Combine ►

◄ **OK to Combine**

Oils and Fats

Butter • Margarine
All oils, including olive,
vegetable, safflower
Avocados • Olives • Coconuts

DO NOT COMBINE FOODS FROM CHART 1 AND 2

CHART 2

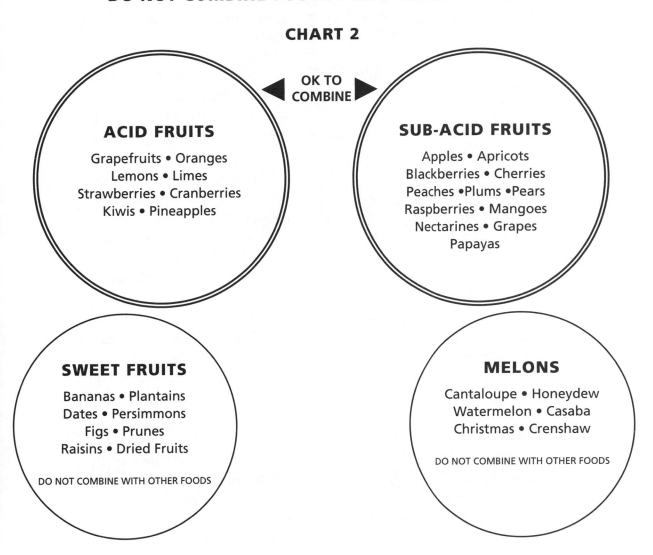

◀ OK TO COMBINE ▶

ACID FRUITS

Grapefruits • Oranges
Lemons • Limes
Strawberries • Cranberries
Kiwis • Pineapples

SUB-ACID FRUITS

Apples • Apricots
Blackberries • Cherries
Peaches • Plums • Pears
Raspberries • Mangoes
Nectarines • Grapes
Papayas

SWEET FRUITS

Bananas • Plantains
Dates • Persimmons
Figs • Prunes
Raisins • Dried Fruits

DO NOT COMBINE WITH OTHER FOODS

MELONS

Cantaloupe • Honeydew
Watermelon • Casaba
Christmas • Crenshaw

DO NOT COMBINE WITH OTHER FOODS

I've been food combining for years, and along the way I've discovered some of my own personal tips that I want to share with you. These are helpful hints that have worked for me, and they might work well for you, too.

For the most part, I divide my day into three food combining segments. I eat fruit in the morning, a protein lunch, and a starch dinner. This gives me a cleansing fruit meal first thing in the morning, my energy-packed protein lunch in the middle of my day, and the slow, steady release of energy from eating complex carbohydrates at night. I can't always keep to this routine (especially if my work schedule prohibits it), but I find that it's what really works best for me and my lifestyle. Sometimes I'll eat my protein lunch in the form of a starch-legume (rice and beans, tofu stir-fry, pasta with lentils, or split pea soup with bread, etc.), which makes a complete protein.

If for some reason you're the kind of person who experiences that after-lunch four o'clock energy slump, try saving some of your lunch to reenergize your batteries. Remember that with food combining, your body will be digesting so efficiently that you may get hungry more often. (That's normal and desirable.) It's better to eat smaller meals more often so as not to overtax your digestive system.

If you miscombine food, there are always ways to offset the bad combination. If you eat a protein with a starch, you can eat some legumes with the starch, and it will "convert" the starch to a complete protein. Let's say you eat chicken with rice for lunch. If you eat some beans (any kind), the chicken-rice combination will digest more easily than if you *don't* eat the beans. If you eat sushi (fish with rice) which is automatically a bad combination, make sure you add either miso soup or edameme (cooked steamed soybeans) to your bill. If beans or soy products aren't available to help round out your miscombined meals, you can always (in a pinch) eat some peanuts after the meal to offset the bad combination. (Peanuts are fattening, I know, but eating a few will make the digestive process more comfortable, and the meal will be less fattening in the long run. This has worked well for me, anyhow.) Speaking of nuts, another good tip is that if you're going to eat a lot of nuts, make sure you eat an acid fruit with them. I really had to figure out this one, because nuts (especially cashews) are one of my favorite indulgences, so when I do eat them, I drink a glass of orange juice or eat some other acid fruit if I can't resist. (You can't imagine how many people I've had to explain this little trick to while sitting next to them on an airplane!)

One of the best things I've ever read about eating is that you should never eat your next meal until you have "resolved" your last meal. What does this mean? After you eat, you should feel satiated and comfortable (like you've just had a tune-up). Hours later, or definitely the next morning, you should feel hungry and ready to eat again. However, if after you eat, you feel stuffed, and the next morning you're still feeling uncomfortable from the heavy meal you ate the night before, you shouldn't wake up and eat a heavy breakfast. If you're still full from lunch (or the food didn't sit well with you), don't eat a big dinner just because it's "dinner time." Knowing certain food combining tips helps you resolve your last meal.

Certain diets purposely miscombine food because they want you to feel somewhat "unresolved." The classic "one bread exchange, one protein exchange, followed by a fruit exchange" approach to dieting was designed to teach people who are used to consuming large amounts of food to eat less by eating smaller portions, and yet they'll still feel full. Mixing starch and protein and topping it off with a fruit will definitely make you feel like you've eaten a bigger meal than you have. Ultimately, these diets tend not to work in the long run because your body never gets to experience that really well-digested, cleaned-out feeling that you start to prefer and strive for.

Some people can tolerate certain bad food combinations better than others can, but at times of illness or detoxification (or getting into shape for that "big" event), it may be more important to adhere to a stricter food combining plan than usual. It's without a doubt the B.E.S.T. way to keep everything flowing and moving through your system.

Even though I do not eat dairy (have I beaten that dead cow enough yet?), I do eat a lot of foods high in calcium, such as broccoli, salmon, figs, oats, green leafy vegetables, sesame seeds, tofu, and blackstrap molasses. Who says you have to drink your milk?

You actually end up consuming less fat when you food combine, because you don't need to differentiate the flavors you're eating. For example, if you eat a piece of bread, you can really taste the bread. If you eat a piece of turkey, you can taste the flavor of the turkey. As soon as you put them together, you need a layer of fat (mayonnaise) to distinguish them! With food combining, you taste the individual foods instead of mixing the foods and flavors together so that you can't tell them apart.

One question I get asked all the time is whether you can drink alcohol while food combining. The answer is yes (in moderation, of course), but there are some guidelines to follow and some drinks that are better than others. One of the reasons Michael Caine liked this way of eating so much is that it's one of the few diets in which you don't have to give up your social life. Drink two glasses of water for every ounce of hard liquor, four ounces of wine, or eight ounces of beer that you drink. When eating starches, it is better to drink beer or grain alcohol (vodka, scotch, etc.), since they are starch-based. Ideally, you should drink wine and champagne only with fruit, which makes sense because champagne and wine are derived from grapes. However, I often drink wine with fish since fish is the most concentrated (yang) food I eat, and wine is the most expansive (yin) thing I consume. They balance each other, and I feel fine from that combination.

Water, of course, is extremely important to your health. Drink only spring or bottled water. If you use ice, it should also come from a pure water source. If you can, try to avoid drinking sparkling or bubbly water since the carbon dioxide gas used to charge the water can interfere with your digestion. Liquids should be consumed fifteen minutes before a meal or one hour after eating. Ideally, you should never drink anything with your meal because it dilutes your digestive juices, thereby interfering with proper digestion. But, if you have to, make sure you sip rather than gulp your drink.

✳ ✳ ✳ ✳ ✳ ✳ ✳ ✳ ✳ ✳

MARILU'S PERSONAL FOOD COMBINING TIPS

1. Divide your day into three food combining segments: preferably eat fruit only in the morning, a protein lunch, and a starch dinner.
2. Some days you may want to eat your protein lunch as a starch-legume meal, which makes a complete protein.
3. If you experience a four o'clock energy slump, try saving some of your lunch to recharge your batteries.
4. If you miscombine by eating starches with protein, eat some legumes with the starch, and the starch will become a complete protein.
5. Never eat nuts without also eating some acid fruit with it.
6. I choose not to eat dairy products, but I do eat foods high in calcium so that I get a sufficient amount of it in my diet.
7. If you do eat dairy, combine it with an acid fruit, especially pineapple, that contains bromelain, an enzyme that helps the stomach digest dairy.
8. When drinking alcohol, follow these rules:
   a. Drink two glasses of water for every one ounce of liquor, four ounces of wine, or eight ounces of beer.
   b. Drink beer and grain alcohol (vodka, scotch, rye whiskey, sake, etc.) when eating starches.
   c. Ideally, you should drink wine and champagne only with fruit.
9. Drink spring or bottled water only.
10. Drink liquids fifteen minutes before eating or one hour after eating.

✳ ✳ ✳ ✳ ✳ ✳ ✳ ✳ ✳ ✳

In 1981, I went to a health spa, The Palms, in Palm Springs, California, with two of my sisters. We had made up our minds that instead of eating the typical spa cuisine (small portions, low-calorie, miscombined food), we were going to eat larger, well-food combined meals the entire week we were there. At the beginning of the week, the other guests looked at what we were eating and shook their heads in total disbelief, as if to say, "No way are those three going to lose weight eating like that!" Even though we ate more food than any of the other guests, by mid-week, we had all lost weight. Everyone at the spa started asking questions about *"our"* diet. By the end of the week, we all looked and felt great, we had vibrant energy (my sister JoAnne lost twelve pounds) and best of all, *we didn't feel deprived*. In fact, the other guests were so inspired by our results, they asked me to lecture about the virtues of food combining.

✳   ✳   ✳   ✳   ✳   ✳   ✳   ✳   ✳   ✳

MARILU'S "FIX IT" CHART
FOR FOOD COMBINING

- If you eat protein and starch during the same meal, eat some legumes.
- If you eat nuts, eat an acid fruit with them.
- If you still eat dairy, make sure to eat an acid fruit.
- If you've overloaded on pasta, eat an apple the next morning.
- If you've eaten too much protein, eat papaya the next morning.
- If you've eaten too much sugar, eat grapes the next morning.
- If you've eaten too much salt, eat watermelon the next morning.

✳   ✳   ✳   ✳   ✳   ✳   ✳   ✳   ✳   ✳

10 | STEP 7: Fat—The Good, the Bad, and the Ugly

FAT OR FICTION?
QUIZ: TEST YOUR FAT IQ

The following quiz is a short probe of your fat IQ. How much do you really know about the food you're eating?

- What is "fat"?

- What is "saturated fat"?

- What is "monounsaturated fat"?

- What is "polyunsaturated fat"?

- Which fat is healthiest?

- What percent of calories consumed is the maximum suggested by experts to be from fat? How about the minimum amount?

- Do you know your blood cholesterol level?

- Is counting fat grams a better way to lose weight than counting calories?

- Have you noticed that you're still hungry after eating fat-free snacks?
- Is butter better for you than margarine?

❋ ❋ ❋ ❋ ❋ ❋ ❋ ❋ ❋ ❋

"Fat-free," "low-fat," and "high-fat" seem to have an overbearing presence in our world. People are fat obsessed, but how well did you do on the above quiz? The type of fat you eat matters. It's impossible (not to mention unhealthy) to try to maintain a "fat-free" lifestyle. While most people know how much they weigh, very few people know their blood cholesterol level. When I first started my program it was around 227. For the last fifteen years, it's been in a healthy range of 140–155. It's an important number to know, because it helps measure your risk for heart disease. A diet high in fat will lead to a higher cholesterol level, making you a candidate for bigger problems later in life. But remember, low fat doesn't mean no fat. Food needs fat to taste good, and quite frankly, our bodies need some fat too.

The Skinny on Fat

Fat in food does do your body some good. It is a necessary nutrient. Fat provides essential fatty acids, from which your body makes molecules it needs to function properly. It acts as a wall of protection around your vital organs like your heart and kidneys. It also acts as an insulator for the body. Fat carries essential (fat-soluble, meaning they dissolve in fat) vitamins A, D, E, and K. These vitamins cannot be absorbed into your body without fat. Although a diet high in fat is unhealthy, fat is the ingredient that makes most foods taste better, because flavor adheres to fat. Fat can offer a concentrated source of energy because fats have a tendency to pack together if they're not in water, so they become a source for greater energy storage. Fat protects your internal organs from going into shock. It insulates the body in extreme temperature conditions. It also acts as an emergency fuel supply in times of illness. Extremely low-fat diets suck the oil right out of your skin. You need a certain amount of fat in your diet for skin to look healthy.

Lexicon of Fats

Diet myths, like "lose thirty pounds in thirty days," or "think yourself thin" are wonderful ideas, but in reality these promises are really just a setup for failure. Eating a diet that is totally "fat-free" falls right into this category of wishful thinking. Fat (which I think is truly just misunderstood) can be your friend.

So, which fats are okay to eat and which ones are not? It's so easy to get confused by all the information (and misinformation) provided to us. For nutritional purposes, fats can be divided into three categories: saturated, monounsaturated, and polyunsaturated, which is based on the amount of hydrogen each one carries. *Saturated* fats have no more room for any additional hydrogen. An easy way to remember what's a saturated fat is to think of animals. All animal fats, such as those found in meat, poultry, dairy products, and eggs, are saturated. Chocolate, coconut oil, and products made with lard are also saturated fats. These are considered the least healthy forms of fat because they are the highest in cholesterol. Saturated fats can also cause the body itself to produce higher levels of cholesterol. *Monounsaturated*

> *A normal-weight adult has around 30 billion fat cells. Someone who gains a large amount of weight, 150 pounds or more, can increase the number of fat cells in his or her body to over 100 billion.*

fats have a little extra room for hydrogen (one more atom) and are somewhat better for you than saturated fats. They are oils like olive, peanut, and canola. Peanut butter and avocados are also monounsaturated fats. People usually think avocados are so fattening, but they're not as bad as you think. They're better than eating a saturated fat. *Polyunsaturated* fats have room for many more hydrogen atoms and are the healthiest form of fat. Corn oil is an example of polyunsaturated fat. Fish, soy, corn, sunflower, and safflower oils are all polyunsaturated fats. English walnuts, salad dressings, mayonnaise, and margarine where liquid oil is the first ingredient are also polyunsaturated. Most experts agree that limiting your daily fat intake to less than 30 percent of total calories consumed is the best approach to eating a healthy diet. Interestingly, your daily percent of total calories consumed should not fall below 15 percent from fat. Of course, to stay within this range of 15–30 percent, you should try to avoid eating saturated fats as much as you can.

> *Americans eat about 125 pounds of fat a year. One out of every four Americans over the age of twenty has an unhealthy level of cholesterol.*

Cholesterol

Cholesterol is the waxy substance that contributes to the formation of many essential compounds, including vitamin D, bile acid, estrogen, and testosterone. (Without cholesterol you would have no sex drive!) Your body actually manufactures all the cholesterol you need (through the liver) and that means that eating fatty foods makes a surplus of the substance. All animal-related foods and drinks contain cholesterol. It's easy to remember which foods have it because they too come from animals that have livers, and therefore they also manufacture cholesterol in their bodies. The American Heart Association recommends that our diets be made up of less than 30 percent of the day's total calories from fat, less than 10 percent from saturated fat, and less than 300 milligrams of dietary cholesterol. Some people are born with a genetic predisposition to having high cholesterol and should be particularly careful in their food choices. Studies show that the more saturated fat and trans-fatty acids (a fat that is made when a liquid fat is turned into a solid fat, like margarine or hydrogenated oils used for cooking) people eat, the higher their cholesterol will be.

> *At age eighteen, my cholesterol was in the 250 range. At twenty-eight, using Mevacor, I was around 200. Today, after six months on Marilu's program, my cholesterol level is 169—without drugs!*
> TERRY WITTER, FRIEND OF MARILU,
> AGE THIRTY-SEVEN

High levels of cholesterol are linked to heart disease as well as cancer. The good news is that you can affect your cholesterol level by changing your diet. Limiting the amount of fat that you eat, increasing foods that are rich in soluble fiber, and staying at a healthy weight are all heart-smart ways to keep your cholesterol under control. Your total blood cholesterol is the amount of cholesterol circulating in your bloodstream. It provides a direct correlation between the amount of plaque deposited in your arteries. It is composed of your HDL (good cholesterol) and LDL (bad cholesterol) levels. Experts agree that your cholesterol level should be below 200, and ideally 100 plus your age. HDL, your white-hat-wearing cholesterol, gets rid of the garbage in your blood. The higher your HDL is, the better off you'll be. LDL, those bad boys of blood, is the cholesterol that builds up on your artery walls and in your system. An easy way to remember the difference is by the first letter. "H" stands for Happy (or Henner!) and "L" stands for Loser!

Nutrients such as lecithin, vitamin E, and vitamin C, as well as niacin, are essential to lowering your cholesterol levels. These nutrients are cleansing to the body, especially your arteries. Soybeans, which I love, are a great source of lecithin, as are most beans. Vitamin C strengthens the walls of your blood vessels. Cabbage, peppers, and citrus fruits are great sources of vitamin C. Plant fiber is also a good way to reduce fat in the blood and helps prevent hardening of the arteries. That's why doctors so often recommend a high-fiber diet. Grains, like rye, quinoa, and oats, are especially good cleansing agents in the body. Unprocessed grains contain niacin and are the best source for vitamin E from their oils.

Twice as many people die from heart and blood vessel disease as from all cancers combined.

It's important to keep your cholesterol level in check because for every 1 percent you lower your cholesterol, you decrease your chance of a heart attack by 2 percent! When plaque builds up on the arteries, it impedes the blood flow through that artery. Plaque is made up of cholesterol, fat, and other debris in the body, and it can grow. As it increases, it blocks the passageways more and more. Keeping your cholesterol level at 150 or below is the heart-smartest way to prevent heart disease.

Limiting—Not Eliminating—Fat

Eating too much fat results in some really harmful consequences. The obvious one is that fat makes you fat. Gram for gram, fat delivers more than twice as many calories as carbohydrates and protein. One gram of fat is equal to nine calories. You have to be really careful with fat-free foods, though, because they tend to be very fattening. Taking the fat out loses the flavor, so food manufacturers compensate by adding other ingredients, like artificial flavorings, sugar, and syrups, all of which are high in calories. Read your food labels! Some fats are definitely easier to spot than others are. Butter, cream cheese, salad dressings, mayonnaise, and cheese are all obvious fat foods. Meats, like sausage, pepperoni, bologna, bacon, corned beef, and hot dogs, aren't so obvious, but they're all high in fat. Ice creams, coleslaw, pasta salads, and potato salad are also high fat. (Of course, these days, there are a lot of low-fat healthy substitutes for these products.)

Even though fat grams are easier to count, calories are what really do you in. Watching the fat in your diet is important, and balancing your intake among fats, protein, and carbohydrates is the best combination for good health.

Trying to eliminate fat from your diet is hardly the answer to better health. Fat, as I said earlier, is essential to your health. The key is to successfully replace the bad fat with good fat. If you let your fat intake fall below 20 percent of your calories from fat a day, you may start eating more volume of food because you'll have a harder time getting full. Fats digest really slowly (much more slowly than carbohydrates and proteins), and they take the longest to exit your body.

Every time you put on weight, your body makes new fat cells. Once these fat cells are made, they stay in your body forever. Every time you lose weight, these fat cells just hang out in your body waiting to get plumped up again. That's why so many people who lose weight on a diet and go back to their old eating habits put on the weight so easily again. When I was at my heaviest (around 170), I made all of those fat cells. They're still there, waiting around to plump up. That's why it would be so much easier for me to get fat again than someone who has never been fat. But it would take a lot for me to get fat again, based on the type of food I eat now. I would have to go back to my old ways of eating, which I could never do. I'm not neurotic about fat because I know and truly understand that we must eat some fat in our diet to stay healthy. I'm just smarter about my choices and sources of fat. It always makes me laugh when someone says she won't eat a cookie but won't hesitate to eat a whole box of fat-free SnackWell's!

Moderation is the key to success. You have to consciously make an effort to reduce your fat intake, but it's not impossible. If you're still eating dairy, choose low-fat dairy products whenever you can. Remove the skin from chicken, and avoid eating the fried version! Trimming the fat around the meat you eat will help cut down on your fat. (It makes sense that you don't want to eat the fat of another animal anyway!) If you do eat meat, try eating lower fat selections. Try substituting turkey for any of your meat needs. It's much lower in fat and can replace meat in almost every recipe. Fish is an excellent source of protein, and there are so many varieties you won't get bored. Use caution when eating pasta, because the sauces can be major culprits of fat. Oil, butter, and dairy-based sauces will sneak up on you and definitely bite you in the butt! If you eat eggs, go for egg whites. The yolk is loaded with cholesterol.

Unfortunately, ice cream is a big, bad, source of high fat and cholesterol, but you don't have to give it up totally. You can try low-fat, or rice or soy ice cream as good low-fat alternatives.

Living a low-fat lifestyle will pave the road for your total health. It's fairly easy these days to maintain that existence, even if you eat out all the time. Most restaurants prepare low-fat, healthy alternatives every day, so there's no excuse!

11 | STEP 8: The Beauty of Exercise and Stress Reduction

*T*hese days, I get most of my exercise dancing eight shows a week in the hit Broadway musical *Chicago*. Still, I look for the time (and actually have the energy) to incorporate other types of exercise into my daily routine. Whether I'm doing Pilates (a form of exercise in which your body fights against the force of gravity, working on an apparatus that has springs), an early-morning stretch, or just dancing around my living room with my sons, Nicky and Joey, for twenty minutes a day, I try to "move" as much as I can.

I know that my final breakthrough in weight loss came once I decided that I would break a sweat for at least twenty minutes every day. I had decided that the gym was too inconvenient and time-consuming and that a personal trainer was way too expensive. (I had been working with a trainer at the time, but when I moved, I was only making it to one out of three weekly sessions, so it just didn't make ene.) All I really needed was to make the time in my schedule to get moving. I would put on a record, the radio, whatever I could find, and just dance and sweat like crazy. I always felt great after those workouts. I started doing this on December 1,

1987, and by Christmas I had lost eight pounds! For years, even though I had been eating as well as I did, those stubborn last ten pounds just wouldn't come off. Breaking a sweat EVERY DAY for at least twenty minutes was the missing piece to the puzzle that I had been trying to solve for years! From that time until now, I have maintained my ideal weight range (except of course, when I was pregnant) without a struggle. Hallelujah! Even if you don't have time to go to the gym, you can get up and dance (even if it's while you're vacuuming or doing laundry!). Put on your favorite CD and jump around and have some fun.

Even though many of you have heard the following information before, I feel it is important to review some of the basics about exercising. For years, it's been proven that your body benefits tremendously from incorporating a regular exercise program into your life. What may be new information to you is how many options are available today. If you have never exercised before (or you're just starting again after being on a hiatus), begin your program slowly. Consult your physician before you start any exercise program. Gradually increase the difficulty of your workouts as your strength and endurance increases. *If exercises are properly performed*, you can not overload your body by exercising. A tip for dressing for your workout: I wear *two* exercise bras for extra support, two pairs of socks for extra cushion, and I put Vaseline on my feet to keep them soft. It also helps reduce any friction that might cause blisters. (Since I'm a dancer, this is especially important for me, because my feet are the tool of my trade!)

It's best if you are working at a level that is even with your abilities. Ideally, you should hit your "target heart rate zone" each time you work out. Your target heart rate zone is 60–80 percent of the maximum number of beats your heart can produce per minute. To see if you're working at the right level, you'll want to work at a level that increases your heart rate to a challenging level but doesn't go beyond that range. If you work below that zone it won't be effective in conditioning your cardiovascular system. To check your heart rate, gently place a finger over the artery in your neck and count the number of beats for ten seconds. Multiply that number by six. This will give you the number of beats per minute.

❋   ❋   ❋   ❋   ❋   ❋   ❋   ❋   ❋   ❋

FINDING YOUR TARGET HEART RATE:

1. Find your resting heart rate by subtracting your age from 220. That number is the absolute maximum level you should ever work at.
2. To find your target *heart* rate range, multiply your maximum heart rate by the percentage you want to work at (60–80 percent).
3. To calculate your target *training* range, divide your training heart rate by six.

For example, if you are forty years old, subtract forty from 220, and your maximum heart rate is 180 beats per minute (bpm). If you work at 60 percent of your maximum, you will have 108/bpm, or eighteen beats per ten seconds. If you work at 80 percent of your maximum, you will have 144 bpm or twenty-four beats per ten seconds. Your target range is eighteen to twenty-four beats per ten seconds. You must work within this range to work most efficiently.

❋   ❋   ❋   ❋   ❋   ❋   ❋   ❋   ❋   ❋

Don't let finding your target heart rate deter you from getting started or scare you like math class. The most important thing is that you GET MOVING! Eventually, as you become better conditioned cardiovascularly, you will find that you'll be working within that zone. The best advice I can give you about exercise is to find something you like doing and DO IT. Don't be afraid to add a little variety into your program. No one says you have to do only one thing. Spice it up! You want to work out at least three days a week for a minimum of twenty minutes to see real results, but I know that aiming for *seven days a week* will get you even further (because then you'll probably do at least five days). Even if on some of those days you only stretch for ten minutes, it's better than doing nothing at all. Make sure you warm up your muscles before doing any kind of exercise, and don't forget to cool down and lower your heart rate after your workout. Stretching *after* you exercise is as important (if not more important) as warming up before. It helps keep your muscles pliable and will reduce muscle soreness later. It's best if you are consistent with your workouts. They're good for the head as well as for the body. Exercising doesn't require an expensive gym membership or lots of fancy equipment. As I mentioned earlier, you can simply choose to just dance around the house. One side of a cassette will do it. I'm sure, however, that if you're deciding to get started on a regular program, you might be a little confused about all your options. You are no longer limited to simply doing old-fashioned calisthenics (although some experts still believe that these are the most effective exercises you can do!). Your form really counts when exercising, so be certain that you are doing it right. Your options are as varied as sneakers these days: aerobics, weight training, kick boxing, yoga, tai chi, walking, running, spinning, stair climbing, even wall climbing! (And if you really want to challenge yourself, try skipping for a mile. If you can do it, drop me a line . . . I'd like to meet you.)

Most gyms offer trainers who can work with you in the beginning stages of your program. It's often a service provided for new members, to better acquaint you with the facility and to show you the ropes. Working out should be a fun experience and not a horrific hour of terror where you feel so intimidated that you do nothing but panic. (Okay, some people can work up a sweat this way, but I don't think it's as much fun!) And hey . . . how 'bout those locker rooms? Do you hate them as much as I do? Small towels, small lockers, and *bad lighting!!!* You've never looked worse when you're trying to look better. It does nothing for your confidence (let alone your complexion), but just know that we *all* feel the same way, so get over it. (Or throw on a coat over your workout clothes and shower at home.)

Like everything we do in life, practice makes perfect! So don't be afraid to make a mistake here and there. It happens to everyone. If you don't know how a machine at the gym works, ask someone. (Safety comes first.) It's a great way to meet new people, and an even better way to stay healthy! You may fumble through those first few aerobics classes, but you'll get the hang of it—I promise.

Simply taking a walk around your neighborhood (some cities even have "mall walks" in local shopping malls) or riding a bicycle with your kids is a great way to get moving. You can even go to your local video store and rent an exercise video (like mine!) and work out with your favorite celebrity or professional trainer right in the privacy of your own home. Of course, if money is no object, you can hire your own personal trainer who comes to your house and brings everything you need to lead you through a safe and effective workout. (This is obviously an expensive option, but if motivation is a problem, it's awfully hard to not work out when you've made an appointment with someone, AND you're paying that person a small fortune!) If you do decide to work out with a trainer (either at your gym or at home), make sure he or she is certified. You want to make sure that trainers know what they're doing so their carelessness doesn't hurt you. Another great alternative to working with a trainer is to find a "workout buddy." Maybe you have a friend who hasn't quite made it to the gym yet, either. Be each other's conscience. Motivate each other to get with the program and start moving your butts! Seeing results together can be a truly gratifying and bonding experience. Besides, misery loves company, right? Healthy competition can be fun, but just don't get *so* competitive that you start derailing each other.

The following chart provides you with the average number of calories used in a one-hour period.

ACTIVITY	CALORIES EXPENDED PER HOUR
Ballroom dancing	330
Bed making	234
Bowling	264
Bricklaying	240
Carpentry	408
Cycling (5.5 mph)	210
Desk work	132
Driving a car	168
Farm work in field	438
Gardening	220
Golf	300
Handball and squash	612
Horseback riding (trot)	480
Ironing (standing up)	252
Lawn mowing (hand mower)	462
Painting at an easel	120
Piano playing	150
Preparing a meal	198
Roller skating	350
Running (10 mph)	900
Scrubbing floors	216
Sitting and eating	84
Sitting and knitting	90
Sitting and reading	72
Skiing	594
Sleeping (basal metabolism)	60
Standing up	138
Sweeping	102
Swimming (leisurely)	300
Tennis	420
Volleyball	350
Walking	216

ACTIVITY	CALORIES EXPENDED PER TEN MINUTES Body Weight in Pounds	
	125	175
Badminton	43	65
Baseball	39	54
Basketball	58	82
Bowling (nonstop)	56	78
Canoeing (4 mph)	90	128
Cycling (5.5 mph)	42	58
Cycling (13 mph)	89	124
Dancing (moderately)	35	48
Dancing (vigorously)	48	66
Football	69	96
Golf	33	48
Horseback riding	56	78
Ping-Pong	32	45
Racquetball	75	104
Running (5.5 mph)	90	125
Running (7 mph)	118	164
Shoveling snow	65	89
Sitting (watching TV)	10	14
Skiing (alpine)	80	112
Skiing (cross-country)	98	138
Skiing (water)	60	88
Squash	75	104
Standing	12	16
Swimming (backstroke)	32	45
Swimming (crawl)	40	56
Tennis	56	80
Volleyball	43	65
Walking (downstairs)	56	78
Walking (upstairs)	146	202
Walking (2 mph)	29	40

Stress—What the Hell Is It and Why Is It Bugging Me?

Stress is different for everyone. A traffic jam, taking a test, your annual review at work, even a blind date (especially a blind date!) can all bring on a stressful response. Have you ever wondered where the word *stress* came from? Whom do we have to thank for coining the phrase *stressed out?* Well, oddly enough, it all started in a science laboratory in the 1930s. A young endocrinologist named Hans Selye (who was a clumsy scientist, to say the least) kept dropping his lab rats and then would chase them around the room until he finally trapped them. He found (through his research) that these rats were so upset about being dropped and trapped, they were developing ulcers and shrunken immune tissue. He was literally making the rats sick by his own ineptness. He searched for a word to describe this reaction to life under severe tension, and came up with "stress," which he borrowed from an engineering term used to define a structure that is in jeopardy of collapse due to an unstable foundation or some other structural flaw.

Life today would be unbearable for those rats. Our schedules are overcommitted and there simply isn't enough time to "get it all in." We work too much, schlep the kids, care for the house, pay the bills, run errands, cook dinner, nurture our family and friends, and when exactly are we supposed to fit in a workout, let alone a little downtime? We're so busy juggling all those balls in the air, we forgot that life doesn't have to be this way at all! All the experts agree that the bulk of the stress in our lives is self-inflicted. We are in control of *most* of those areas in our lives that somehow bring on stress. It's our attitude about *dealing* with them that creates the level of stress in our lives. Striking the right balance in life is the key to eliminating tension and stress. I know . . . easier said than done.

The Effects of Stress on Your Body

The way our bodies physically respond to stress is preprogrammed. It is actually genetically passed down from generation to generation. When the senses perceive any threat to our existence, the brain triggers a flood of chemicals throughout the body that help prepare us for our response. You may have heard of "fight or flight" response, which is an ancient survival mechanism and is chemically the same type of response as modern stress. Stress can also be an asset under the right circumstances. When we sense a dangerous situation, our bodies release adrenaline and other chemicals that make us more alert, raise our blood pressure, and increase our strength, speed, and reaction time. In circumstances where there is an actual physical danger threatening us, this is an ideal response. The problem is that the body cannot differentiate between a physical threat and a mental threat, so it responds the same way in either circumstance. That's when stress can become harmful to your health. The chemicals that are released can linger in your bloodstream because you don't burn them off. Stress can manifest itself in your body in a wide variety of ways. Some side effects, which seem slight and insignificant at the time, can in fact develop into much larger problems, and if left untreated will continue to persist. Heart disease, high blood pressure, weight loss or gain, cancer, and depression are all linked to stress. Other symptoms, such as hair loss, fatigue, a change in your complexion, insomnia, a low libido, and a disruption of your menstrual cycle are also associated with stress.

Studies show that stress can significantly reduce the power of our immune systems by inhibiting the disease-fighting cells in the bloodstream, especially as women grow older and stop producing estrogen, which blocks the buildup of plaque in the arteries. Stress increases heart rate and blood pressure, which change the inner lining of the blood vessels, making it much easier for blood to clot. Stress can also affect the way our bodies deal with cholesterol, which can also increase the formation of plaque.

Reducing Stress in Your Life

The first step in reducing stress is usually to identify those areas in your life that are causing it. (Don't let this stress you out! Reducing stress shouldn't be stress-inducing.) But understand this: *Everything in life causes stress.* It's your attitude and approach that can make the difference between waking up and facing your day with hopeful anticipation or dreaded resignation.

The people I know who handle stress well live a far more balanced life than those who just can't seem to cope. The secret seems to be *resilience*, an ability to roll with the punches, and to learn how to maneuver life's curves. (I always say the key to your life is how well you deal with Plan B.)

Different things cause stress for different people. For some, the thought of getting up on stage and performing in front of an audience would be a terrifying proposition. Likewise, I wouldn't be able to handle the idea of working as a flight attendant because I would find flying daily so disconcerting.

Pregnant women under stress are approximately one and a half times more likely to give birth prematurely than pregnant women under little or no stress.

Identifying those areas in your life that cause stress is just part of the solution, but it's not the answer. Let's face it, we're never going to completely rid our lives of stress anyway, but *organization* is one of the best ways to alleviate the day-to-day stress. For some of us, reducing stress might require making a list of the things that aggravate us (remember the TBM list from Chapter 3?). Include in another list the things in your life that are making you happy and content (the "Good Nails" list!). Making this list will help you prioritize what needs to be handled, and identify your strengths to handle them. Sometimes seeing these lists side by side will help you understand what hidden tools you might possess that can help you resolve some of the problems (e.g., somewhere on that list of good friends, you might find a good dieting partner, mother's helper, or even a decent divorce lawyer!).

Personally, whenever I have to tackle some huge task, I always say to myself, "Do something small to make yourself feel better." Regardless of how big and daunting the task may be, I may start with something less important from my "to do" list. Completing one small task well (even something as mundane and ridiculous as cleaning my room or organizing my sock drawer) will put me in the "winning syndrome" mode to build up to that much larger task at hand.

Of course, some things in life aren't that easy to just jot down and change, but you might find that seeing things in black and white might help you acknowledge those problems from a new and primed perspective.

A 1994 Gallup Organization Survey on stress and its causes showed that the greatest amount of stress in a person's life (71 percent) is caused by his or her work. (Though many people

> *Four out of every ten American adults say stress is a frequent part of their lives. Stress-related symptoms now account for 90 percent of all visits to a primary care physician, according to the American Institute of Stress in Yonkers, New York.*

said that they felt their *boss* or *the pressure of meeting a deadline* was the cause of their stress.) People stayed late when they didn't have to and came in on weekends when it wasn't required. When further asked about their working conditions, most people actually self-imposed their own deadlines and expectations to meet, thus being the cause of their own stress. Other major areas of stress were (in order) money problems (63 percent), family (44 percent), housework (37 percent), health problems (35 percent), and child care (20 percent). Men and women were surprisingly equal in their concerns over family and housework, though women were more stressed out over child care.

Many people who have a strong reaction to stressful situations are often victims of self-destructive thinking. We must learn not to be our own worst enemies, but rather our own best friends. People who are pessimistic and who are going around always assuming the worst are good examples of this type of behavior. These are people who always know how *everyone else* is feeling and what they're thinking, and it's never good. Someone doesn't return your call for a week, and you instantly think it's because of *you*. (Forget that they might be busy, sick, or on vacation.) Everything is taken as what psychologists refer to as a "narcissistic injury."

> *Adults who live in the western part of the United States are the most stressed out. Southerners are the least stressed out. Adults over the age of fifty-five are less stressed out than younger Americans.*

Despite what you might think, things are rarely as bad as you thought. Try not to get trapped in this "all or nothing" way of thinking. No single episode defines a person, place, or relationship. A bad day at work doesn't mean your job stinks. It means you had a bad day at work, and guess what? We all have those days! It's no reason to beat yourself up (or anyone else, for that matter!).

Another way to bring on unnecessary stress is to assume responsibility for something that is beyond your control. This can range from taking personally anything anyone says to you to feeling like you're solely responsible for everyone else's "good time" to not knowing how to delegate because you're the *only* one who knows how to do anything right. (Some of the people I know who do that are closet "control freaks" who like to think of themselves as personally responsible for everything that happens.)

Exercise

In my opinion, exercise is one of the greatest outlets to relieve stress. Regular aerobic workouts reduce stress more effectively than any medication, psychiatric intervention, biofeedback, and conventional stress management, according to David S. Holmes, Ph.D., professor of psychology at the University of Kansas in Lawrence. Exercise can help burn off those stress-related chemicals that are lingering in our bloodstreams. Working out also releases endorphins into our systems that relax the mind. Of course, the physical benefits to working out are always a great reason to stay on an exercise program. Research shows that thirty minutes of intense aerobic exercise immediately reduces tension in the body.

Relaxation exercise is another alternative to reducing stress and letting go of tension. Meditation, yoga, tai chi, or even deep breathing can all relax the mind, body, and spirit. I often find that any of these are reenergizing and help restore a calm, less-stressed atmosphere. The best part of any of these exercises is that you can practice them anytime, anywhere. You just need to make a little time to do them. Practicing anything that calms the mind and opens your soul is a positive addition to anyone's day. If you've never tried these forms of exercise, there are lots of books available and most health clubs around the country are offering classes these days.

Just Say NO!

Sometimes, stress can be alleviated by saying one simple word: "no." I always refer to November as the month of "no" because you have to say "yes" to everything in December. (I remind myself of this by saying the first two letters are "N-O.") I think that, in general, people don't always say "no" when they really want to. They say "yes" to dinners when they'd rather be home in bed reading a good book, or they sacrifice their personal time under the guise of doing nice things for other people, when all it's really doing is helping them avoid taking care of themselves (like working out). Learning to say "no" will greatly help diminish the level of stress in your life, and there are graceful ways to get out of doing something, especially if you don't want to. Learning how to manage your time and your life effectively will definitely reduce stress. It's nice to be needed in life, but not at the expense of our health, our happiness, or our sanity.

Laughter Is the Best Medicine

Laughing is one of the best ways to beat stress that I know of, and definitely one of the most fun. There are laughing clubs in India whose members claim that laughing lowers their blood pressure, revs up their immune system, and actually helps them sleep better at night. A study at Loma Linda University showed that laughing increases various measures of the immune system. It activates T-cells primed to battle infection (natural killer cells that fight tumors and microbes), immunoglobulin A antibodies (which patrol the respiratory tract), and gamma interferon (a key immune system messenger). The levels of cortisol (a hormone that suppresses the immune system) were also significantly lowered. In a nutshell, laughter is the opposite of stress in terms of its effect on the body. (This is a terrific example of the yin and yang philosophy discussed in Chapter 2.)

> *The number of times per day an average preschooler laughs—400. The average number of times per day an average adult laughs—fifteen.*

The greatest benefit of laughter comes in having a sense of humor about the ironies of life. If you can laugh, you can get through anything. It is impossible to laugh and be stressed out at the same time. Laughing is a coping mechanism that acts as a buffer between your immune system and the situation that's causing the stress.

> *It takes seventeen muscles to smile and forty-three to frown.*

Stress and Eating

Some people have a tendency to eat as a result of stress. You have to learn how to manage your mood without food, but for those of you who can't, making the right choices will help reduce stress (not to mention calories!). Three mood-altering neurotransmitters produced by our brains are chemicals designed to pass information from brain cell to brain cell: dopamine, norepinephrine, and serotonin. Dopamine and norepinephrine are energizers. Your brain manufactures them from the amino acid tyrosine, which is found in protein foods. Serotonin acts as either a tranquilizer or an aid in concentration. Carbohydrates encourage serotonin by increasing the brain's supply of the amino acid tryptophan. You can create a certain chemical response to counter the effects of stress by choosing the right foods to eat under stressful circumstances.

If you know you're going to be in a stressful situation, you need to be alert, fast thinking, and not nervous. So it makes sense that you should eat foods that won't have the opposite effect, right? A well-combined fruits-only or carbohydrate-only or protein-only meal eaten before that big meeting or speech is the best choice. Try not to drink a lot of caffeine, as it can add to your nerves. And definitely no sugar! The temporary high will make you feel good, but halfway through that presentation you're going to come crashing down. (How embarrassing it will be when your head hits the table!) But make sure you eat something. Trying to perform on an empty stomach is distracting (not only to you, but imagine someone hearing that loud rumble from your tummy!). Also, sometimes a combination of hunger and tension can result in nausea or a really bad headache.

Nature has a way of guiding us toward making the right choices when we are being tested, and stress is a perfect example. Eating the right food at the right time in the right amount is as effective as taking a tranquilizer, and better for you, too. For this to really work for you, though, you should already be following a balanced eating program. My food combining methods work really well for stress, because there's no undue pressure put on the digestive system. Staying away from fat-laden foods is also a good idea for optimum results. Fat slows down digestion, and serotonin can't be produced in the brain until digestion has taken place. Ideally, you want to eat carbohydrates that break down quickly in the body, and that activate the production of serotonin. Eating something like a bowl of oatmeal or whole grain toast can help.

Some people crave sweets when they're under pressure. (It's that yin and yang thing again. Stress is yang and sweets are yin.) Make sure you don't wolf down your snack, and don't overeat. The only thing you'll get from that is a stomachache and unnecessary extra calories. Your body knows what it needs to get the response you're looking for. You can get results within twenty minutes if you follow these guidelines, and you'll be less wired, worried, and stressed.

Baths and More

Other "stressbusters," such as taking a bath, having a massage, and even just taking fifteen minutes to yourself to do nothing, are all great ways to come back down after a high-intensity situation. Taking a bath can be a wonderful gift. The warmth of the water actually helps restore circulation that the stress and tension reduced. The heated water covers a greater area of your body and helps dilate your blood vessels. A bath allows you to be in a reclining position, so the muscles in your feet, legs, and back can get a rest, too. A bath also allows you to be a little more self-indulgent and selfish because you can pamper yourself with aromatic soaps, candles, and bath oils. These types of bath products disperse evenly in bath water, so more of your body is in continuous contact with the moisturizers and other therapeutic ingredients. They leave you feeling euphoric, relaxed, and rejuvenated.

There are specific techniques to getting the most out of your bath time and to relieving different types of tension. For frazzled nerves, try taking a ten- to twenty-minute bath in very warm water (which will dilate your blood vessels and help you feel calm). Add bath teas, salts, or soaks, infused with geranium, lavender, or seaweed. Bubbles aren't a good idea for the best therapy here, because you really want to reap the benefits of the aromatherapy aspects of the added scents.

Aching muscles can be helped by taking a very warm bath infused with salts (which help draw out lactic acid from the sore muscles) or oils such as peppermint, primrose, or cypress. When I'm feeling like I've done too much and need a break (especially after a two-show day) I really appreciate the benefits of taking a good old-fashioned Epsom salts bath. You should soak for fifteen to twenty minutes for the best results.

If you are exhausted, and can go to bed immediately after taking your bath, soak for ten to fifteen minutes in a bath that has bubbles or oils infused with sleep-inducing elements such as lavender, chamomile, or rose oil. If you need to rejuvenate, take a lukewarm bath and scrub your body all over to wake yourself up. Try using oils with citrus, peppermint, or eucalyptus.

Finally, if you have a sore neck or back (which I often do now that I live in New York; I have to carry everything in a big bag) try taking a hot bath and add to it gels or oils that contain menthol, eucalyptus, juniper, peppermint, or lavender. Take an extra towel and soak it in the water. Add some extra gel to it, roll it up like a compress, and put it around your neck or behind your back. I find this really therapeutic and very calming.

Having a massage is often thought of as something you do only on vacation or as a special treat for yourself every now and then. But studies show that therapeutic massage is very helpful in reducing stress and keeping your body healthy. There are many different types of massage, but a relaxing Swedish massage is probably the best choice for reducing stress. It also promotes relaxation and circulation. It involves long strokes and kneading on bare skin, usually using massage oil that might have some aromatherapy benefit as well. A massage doesn't have to take long, either. You can stop in to almost any salon these days and get a fifteen-minute "pick-me-up" or do some relaxing technique on yourself. You can rub the back of your neck and relieve tension and stress in just a few minutes.

Skin Brushing—
Giving Your Body the Big Brush-off

When you think about what the body is actually eliminating on a daily basis, it makes perfect sense that the elements such as uric acid crystals, catarrh, and other acids can be more easily shed if the top layer of your dead skin is removed. In a way, the skin is similar in function to the kidneys, because it helps us get rid of unwanted and unnecessary uric acids.

Think of your skin like a thin layer of dough that surrounds your body. Even though it weighs twice as much as the liver or the brain, it receives only a third of the blood that circulates throughout your body. Clothes prevent the skin from being able to breathe, as it should. In fact, we don't even sweat like we were meant to. Wearing synthetic fibers, like polyester and nylon, prevents proper perspiration. Natural fabrics like cotton help absorb toxins and waste material being eliminated from the skin. All of this stagnant behavior to our skin increases the need and importance of body brushing. The skin becomes inactive and cannot properly be used as a source of elimination as it should. Skin brushing also helps your body along in the middle of a healing crisis. There isn't a soap available to cleanse your skin as well as skin brushing can. We make new skin every twenty-four hours, so removing the top layer of dead tissue

> *The skin eliminates two pounds of toxic waste each day.*

and cells to expose the healthy lively layer of skin beneath that is the best body cleansing available.

How to Skin Brush

Skin brushing is very simple, and I start my day every morning by using a natural bristle brush that looks like a shoe shining brush. (Make sure you use only a natural bristle, because synthetic fibers such as nylon will irritate your skin.) You want to brush your *dry* skin in an elongated upward motion toward the heart for two to three minutes every morning. (Brushing wet skin can pull or sag your skin and defeat the purpose of removing that dead, dry outer layer.) Start with your feet and ankles, and work your way up the body to your calves and thighs. (I especially love brushing the soles of my feet). Really concentrate on brushing the lymphatic areas of your body (the backs of your knees, your inner thighs, and under your arms) to stimulate those glands and get them started on flushing out those toxins. Brush each arm and hand. Gently brush up your stomach and tush, shoulders and back. Finish this regimen by making sure you cover the entire surface of your body, *excluding* your breasts and face. The brushing should not irritate you. It may take a couple of days to get used to it, but if you hang in there, I promise you will feel the difference in your skin in less than a week.

Skin brushing also helps reduce cellulite, aids in the digestive process, tightens the skin, and stimulates the lymph glands to help the body perform at its peak level. I skin brush before working out so that I sweat evenly all over. Too many people sweat only under their arms and from their faces during a workout. Skin brushing really opens your pores and allows your body to sweat evenly all over, which releases all those toxins from every area of your body. On mornings that I don't work out, I skin brush before I take a shower so that I can rinse the excess residue off my body.

You should use a special soft brush designed for your face if you are going to brush it. These brushes can be easily found in most health food stores. A loofah face sponge works in a similar way, and you can easily get a loofah at most cosmetic or drugstores.

The best way to understand the benefits of skin brushing is to experience it firsthand. Most people find that it feels great, helps keep their skin younger-looking and more vibrant, and actually improves the overall beauty and health of the body. Dry skin brushing is one of the most powerful gifts you can give yourself, your skin, and your lymphatic system on a daily basis. Go ahead and give yourself the big brush-off. You'll be glad you did!

12 | STEP 9: Sleep— The Cure-all

*T*he most common question I am asked about my hectic and crazy schedule is "How do you do it? You never seem tired, yet you keep a schedule that would kill most people. What's your secret?"

I usually tell people about my ten-step program (I'm always looking for converts), but there is no doubt in my mind that none of these steps would make a difference if I didn't reinforce them with a good night's sleep. When I started to read about macrobiotics, one of the first things I grasped on to was that it was unlike other diets or books I read about health that encouraged getting eight hours of sleep a night. Macrobiotics takes the stand that someone who is in good health will need only six hours of sleep a night. Reading this made me feel vindicated and understood because I had spent so many years defending my position that while sleep is unquestionably *essential* to your health, you don't need as much sleep as you think you do. Just as with food, if you improve the quality, the quantity will take care of itself.

Sleep is the one step in my program that is absolutely essential to helping every other step work effectively. I've never been able to handle a problem, thwart a cold, or solve a beauty drama without a good night's sleep. Sleep is the fountain of youth. If someone told you that you could look younger, feel better, boost your energy level, and keep yourself healthy, wouldn't you want to know how to do that? It's simple, it's cheap, and it's as easy as getting a good night's sleep. Your body has a built-in clock that knows when you are sleep-deprived and when you are right on schedule. You can't cheat your need for sleep without cheating yourself. According to Michael Vitiello, Ph.D., associate director of the Sleep and Aging Research program at the University of Washington, Seattle, "Sleep is a part of the constellation of behaviors that maximizes the quality of our lives." It's a pretty safe bet to say that when you sleep better, you feel better. I know that on nights when I have a great night's sleep, I have boundless energy and vitality throughout my entire day. I feel better, and I know that I look healthier, too. On mornings after I haven't had a good night's sleep, I look in the mirror and see the blueprint of my future. (There it is, mapped out on my face). We all know what people who are sleep-deprived look like. They have dark circles under their eyes, their complexions are pale, they have a dazed and spaced-out expression, and they're usually pretty cranky. Their posture is slouchy, their energy level is barely measurable, and they practically slur when speaking. People who are getting enough sleep (and good-quality sleep) can reverse every single one of these side effects caused by sleep deprivation.

What Is Sleep?

Almost all animals on earth have the need for sleep. The exceptions are those creatures lacking complex mental functions, like jellyfish and flatworms. The need for sleep increases as the brain becomes more complicated and as vision plays an increasingly important role in the life of the animal. In people, an internal clock regulates the sleep-wake cycle, which is a small cluster of cells at the back of the brain that governs the release of hormones that cause drowsiness. Light seems to have a large effect on the sleep-wake cycle, which is why humans tend to sleep at night and are more alert during the day. Once asleep, we go through five stages. Stages one through three occur during light sleep. Stage four, known as delta sleep, represents our deepest sleep. The fifth stage is a state akin to the fight-or-flight response to danger, and kicks into high gear during the REM (rapid eye movement) phase of sleep. This is the "dream" phase of sleep, which is not especially restful or deep. The eyes dart back and forth, and the heart rate and respiration can increase and fluctuate. Large muscles in the body can actually become paralyzed, most likely so that we don't hurt ourselves by thrashing around during our dreams. The deepest and most restful period of sleep is the non-REM phase, during which the heart rate, respiration, and brain waves slow way down. This period of time accounts for 75 percent of sleep for most adults. Adequate delta and REM sleep is essential for good health. Without it, not only do we feel lousy, but also our abilities to learn, memorize, and reason are greatly impaired. (Plus it is also very important for our mental health to be able to dream.)

The Body's Need to Sleep

Scientists know that the body releases its greatest concentration of human growth hormones (HGH) during sleep. These are the main ingredients that help the body repair damaged tissue. HGH spurs cell division and organ growth, particularly during childhood. It tapers off in adults after age thirty. In tests done on animals, severely sleep-deprived subjects suffer a complete breakdown in their vital functions. A study done at the University of Chicago kept lab rats awake for seventeen days. After about a week of enforced consciousness, the rats began to show signs of the strain. Odd lesions began to appear on their tails and paws. They became irritable and they were unable to stabilize their body temperature to make themselves warmer. They ate twice as much as usual, but lost 10–15 percent of their body weight. After seventeen days, the rats died.

There are lots of theories on why our body needs to sleep, but most of these theories are just plain common sense. We function better (like the animal we were meant to be) when we are properly rested. We can't afford to be active twenty-four hours a day. Evolution (and the laws of the universe) dictates that we take a daily period of hibernation, known as sleep. Aristotle believed that sleep was caused by warm vapors coming from the stomach. That was his explanation for why people get sleepy after eating. (I guess Aristotle didn't know about bad food combining.) Another popular theory is that sleep kept us out of harm's way from dangerous predators during the night. There are enough theories on *why* we need sleep to keep you up at night. What experts know is that sleep does have an effect on our health. Get enough sleep, and the effect is positive. Deprive yourself of sleep, and the effects are negative. It's that simple.

Sleep and the Immune System

Like those lab rats, all animals, including humans, cannot survive for very long without sleep. Long-term sleep deprivation can cause fatal blood infections. The immune system begins to fail, and bacteria that we could normally fight off begin to run wild, and because of the weakened immune system, we are unable to effectively fight off disease. *One single night* of sleep deprivation can result in *a 30 percent* decrease in the activity of cells that attack tumors in the human body. When your doctor tells you to "go home and get into bed" or "get some rest" what he or she is really telling you is rest and sleep is a natural way for our body to heal itself.

Sleep and the Brain

Most sleep specialists agree that the mind benefits equally from a good night's sleep. If you're not getting enough sleep, your mind is like scrambled eggs (or tofu). Your memory and cognitive thinking skills lapse, and you feel lethargic, lazy, irritable, and moody. Your ability to concentrate and make sound decisions is paralyzed. All areas of your life are obviously affected by these kinds of sleep-deprivation side effects. Your performance at work and your ability to function in a safe manner are often visible signs of being in a state of sleep deprivation. Traffic accidents, mishaps at the office, or even worse industrial accidents are all commonly linked to lack of sleep. I had the worst car accident of my life as I was driving all night from Chicago on my way to Washington, D.C. Right outside Harrisburg, Pennsylvania, I started to nod out, and awoke when my car drove over the middle barrier, knocking down two reflectors (which I now own because I had to pay for them), landing perpendicular to oncoming traffic. Luckily, no one was hurt and there was no traffic coming toward us. I never again drove when I was tired.

Forty years ago, researchers believed that when we slept, we were giving our brain a "rest." Today, studies show that our brain is actually very hard at work, sparking nerve networks within the body that aren't being exercised during the day. After we're born, sleep seems to activate the immune system. In the womb, sleep allows the brain to develop and stay sharp, say the experts. Sleep serves as a time when the brain can do a "systems check" on the body and all its functions.

Sleep helps the brain develop and mature. It also helps consolidate memory, which probably explains why we become forgetful when we don't get enough sleep. Think of your brain as a cluttered desktop. At the end of the day, it needs to file away the mess so that the next morning you've got some sense of order to start your day. It sorts through new information and old information and formulates an overall perspective for you to work with. That's how we retain information we gather each day, and are able to recall it thereafter. The best time for me to memorize a script is right before I go to bed. I do a quick review of the script in the morning, and I feel totally prepared. If I don't follow this routine, I don't feel I know my lines as well because I haven't "slept" on them.

Insomnia

The first time I experienced insomnia was the night before my first Holy Communion, when I was seven years old. I remember lying in bed, filled with excitement and anticipation about my big day ahead. My heart was beating, my mind was racing, and I just couldn't fall asleep. This has happened to me so many times in my life since then (and for me it's usually connected to anticipation or anxiety), and as I get a little older, I find that it's a little harder to bounce back from a bad night's sleep. Of course, motherhood also enlightened me to never take sleep for granted! Once I became a mom, getting a good night's sleep became so vital that as soon as my head hits the pillow I'm out!

It is said that as we age, our bodies need less sleep. Insomnia (not being able to sleep) is a major problem. It affects nearly twice as many women as men. Two-thirds of the people over age fifty who visit sleep clinics are suffering from some form of insomnia. It's interesting to note that insomnia is not just the inability to fall asleep. There are various kinds of insomnia. "Sleep onset" insomnia is the inability to doze off, and is usually related to stress and anxiety. "Sleep maintenance" insomnia is described as having trouble staying asleep. This is often due to depression, chronic pain, illness, or a disruption in your normal sleep pattern and schedule. Insomnia can last from one night to several weeks (or longer in times of real crises). For women, sleep patterns can fluctuate according to different points in the menstrual cycle. The likelihood of a woman not being able to sleep is highest right before the onset of her menstruation (called "cyclic insomnia"). Insomnia is often linked to PMS, too. The good news is that for most people, once life gets back to normal, their sleeping habits ought to do the same.

There are several solutions to insomnia. Trying to regulate your sleeping habits is a good starting point if it's possible. I know that everyone's schedule varies, but trying to maintain a bedtime as adults is as important as it is for children. You want to make sure that you create a good environment that promotes a comfortable, cozy night's sleep. A dark, quiet, and well-ventilated room is ideal. The bedroom was designed for two purposes. One is to sleep; the other, to have sex. For many people, however, the bedroom has become a place where you read, watch TV, or even work. Training your body to think of that space as the place where you *only* sleep (or have sex) will help it have a natural response when you climb into bed. If you find yourself tossing and turning, get out of bed and do something until you get sleepy. Experts agree that lying awake in bed can add to your insomnia. If you find that you're having no problem falling asleep, but you're waking up too early or in the middle of the night, try pushing your bedtime back a few hours. So, if you normally go to bed around ten and you're awakening in the early morning hours (between three-thirty and five A.M.), try going to bed a little later to offset the early rising. Try not to eat meals (especially protein meals) late at night if you're having problems sleeping. You also want to avoid anything that has caffeine. Alcohol and even nicotine can interrupt your good night's sleep, so you want to try to curtail drinking and smoking at least three hours before you go to bed. Smoking shouldn't be done at any time.

Exercising regularly has been linked to helping people sleep better at night, and many experts think it's the best solution to sleep problems. A recent Stanford University study showed that people with moderate insomnia fell asleep twice as fast and slept an extra hour once they began going for brisk walks. People who do not work their muscles with any regularity are the least likely to be able to get into a full state of relaxation at night. Experts find that a late-afternoon workout helps promote drowsiness at night, but recommend working out any time of the day over no exercise at all. Some people find that working out in the evenings has an adverse affect on their ability to fall asleep, so you might want to avoid working out right before bedtime. (Of course, I need a few hours myself to come down from the energy I have after performing live theater every night, so that explains why I don't go right to bed after my show.)

Don't get dependent on prescription sleeping pills or over-the-counter sedatives. Natural remedies can help induce sleep, and they're not addictive or habit-forming. Experts are finding that people who regularly take sleeping pills are not solving the issue of *why* they're not sleeping. They're merely inducing a state of sleep through ingesting a chemical. Sleeping pills are another question of risk versus benefit. Many people suffer from a sleeping pill hangover the next day, which are often similar to the effects of not sleeping at all. Of course, the issue of addiction is always a major concern. Learning how to adjust your need for sleep can be done naturally and without any side effects.

Natural Remedies

Many natural sedatives found in herbs have been shown to help induce sleep. Everything from chamomile tea to exotic passion-flower extract is easily available. The most effective herb is a valerian extract, which can be found in pill form and tinctures. It can be added to brewed tea, which is recommended because some people think it has an icky taste. A recent study in Chicago showed that of the 128 people researched, all of them who took the herb fell asleep, dropped off faster, and stayed asleep longer. Melatonin has been a real buzzword in recent years. It is a hormone naturally produced by the body that keeps the internal clock in sync with the cycles of day and night. Melatonin (which also comes in pill form) is often used to help induce sleep and is most effective as a short-term solution. Researchers have found that melatonin can help the symptoms brought on by jet lag, which is how it became a popular sleep aid in recent years.

To Nap or Not to Nap—That Is the Question

Some experts argue that taking a mid-afternoon nap will prevent you from having a good night's sleep. Others say that taking that nap is the perfect solution to reviving and refreshing yourself for the rest of your day. It brings back your sharpness and vitality, and can leave you feeling invigorated. I myself am not a regular napper; however, if I'm really tired and need to refresh myself, I have no trouble taking a twenty-minute nap and waking up feeling like I just had a good night's sleep.

TO NAP. Most people, if they take a nap, need around twenty minutes to gain the best benefits of the nap. Anything less is likely to leave you feeling groggier than you did before. The timing of when you take a nap is also important. An afternoon nap is more efficient for the body than a morning nap. You're more likely to feel the need for a nap in the afternoon, as a lot of people get that after-lunch slump caused naturally by your circadian rhythms or, more than likely, by what you ate. A one-hour nap in the afternoon can actually mirror the pattern of a perfect night's sleep. You'll likely cycle through all five stages of sleep, leaving you feeling bright-eyed and bushy-tailed. Morning naps tend to allow you to reach only that restless REM sleep, which is usually what you awoke from earlier that morning.

OR NOT TO NAP. If you are suffering from insomnia, most experts agree that you should try to avoid taking a nap. It can (and usually will) worsen your ability to sleep at night. Many people suffer from sleep inertia (that groggy feeling), which can linger for hours after an afternoon nap. Some people are just not good nappers, and therefore shouldn't take them.

Keeping a Sleep Journal

One of the best ways to track your patterns of sleep is to keep a sleep journal. Keeping track of everything that might be affecting your sleep will help you determine how to get a better night's snooze. Keep a notebook beside your bed and write down what time you went to bed, the number of times you woke up during the night, if you go to the bathroom, or *other* activities.

If you're a woman, keep track of your menstrual cycle, including the first and last day of your period and any symptoms or difficulties. Write down whether you were sleepy the next day, if you took a nap, and keep track of the areas that might be causing you excessive stress. A late-night meal or a few extra glasses of wine are bound to affect your sleep. Keep track of these events so that you can really help yourself get a good night's sleep. Plan on keeping this journal for at least three months so that you can go through it and detect "fixable" patterns. For example, if you find that you are suffering insomnia around the same time every month, you can determine that it is cyclical insomnia and not a more serious chronic problem. You can then take steps to prevent the onset by helping to stabilize your hormone levels with vitamins like B6, and a calcium and magnesium combination.

❋　❋　❋　❋　❋　❋　❋　❋　❋　❋

YOUR SLEEP JOURNAL

- Time you went to bed.
- Number of times you wake during the night (bathroom or "other" activity if any).
- First and last day of your period and any symptoms or difficulties.
- Were you sleepy the next day?
- Did you take a nap during the day?

- Track areas causing excessive stress.
- Keep the journal for at least three months.

❋ ❋ ❋ ❋ ❋ ❋ ❋ ❋ ❋ ❋

Sleep on This

Getting enough sleep allows your body to be a natural healer for almost every ailment that can affect you. It's no wonder people who are totally sleep-deprived find themselves down for the count. They literally work themselves into the ground until their bodies give them a reminder to slow down and get essential rest. Sleep is truly one of the greatest gifts you can give yourself. Your body will thank you, your mind will thank you, and everyone in your life will thank you, too—because you won't be crabby! Zzzzz.

13 | STEP 10: Gusto—The Missing Ingredient in the Mind/Body Connection

*Y*ears ago, my girlfriend Cynthia called me to come to her house to help her get ready for a big skiing weekend with a new boyfriend. It was to be their first romantic weekend together, and she really wanted to look great. She had borrowed several expensive coats from her mother, and wanted me to help her choose which one looked best. She tried on the first coat, walked around in it, all slouchy and self-conscious. The coat hung on her with absolutely no energy and style. My friend Cynthia, who's really beautiful, asked, "Does this look good?" Coat after coat, she looked uncomfortable and ill-at-ease. Finally, after she agonized over each coat, I said to her, "It's not the coats, Cynthia, it's you!" I grabbed a coat, put it on, threw my head back, and walked around like I loved that coat. She said, "That looks great on you!" I explained to her, "It can look great on you, too, but you have to 'work the coat'!" This expression, "work the coat," has taken on great meaning around my friends and family. It has become our slogan for attitude and presentation. It explains that energy that someone has, that enthusiasm for life, that joie de vivre.

That is gusto.

And it has *nothing* to do with looks. Many beautiful people don't have a clue about gusto. Likewise, someone with gusto becomes far more attractive. Gusto is what separates the people in life who are truly successful and enviable.

> *Gusto is feeling great about who you are and what you're doing*
> *no matter what or where you might be.*
>
> LORIN JOSEPH HENNER

Without gusto, you're merely marking time, and with it, you're devouring time and space. People with gusto have that look of vibrant health and carry themselves with confidence and self-assuredness. They have that light behind their eyes, and you can't help but find yourself drawn to someone with that kind of magnetism. I'm not saying that you should go through life carefree and wearing rose-colored glasses. Life is filled with challenges, changes, surprises, and curves. When we are confused or when we take a wrong turn, we may need some help working through the muddle and getting back on track. It is during these times especially that we must believe in ourselves and trust that we can indeed do what we set out to do.

I have found that in life, attitude is everything. My philosophy has always been, "The key to your life is how well you deal with Plan B." Resilience, and the ability to get over things and move on, is everything. To be able to ride the roller coaster of life and *still* want to put your hands in the air with joy and excitement every day is the greatest gift to be honored and envied. So many people are afraid of making a mistake that they stay at zero on the number line. They're so afraid of "minus" that they never get to "plus." Sometimes you have to risk being bad (or embarrassing) to get to good. Ask anyone who's taken up a musical instrument, or singing, or dancing. (Or, better yet, ask anyone who has to listen to anyone who's taken up a musical instrument, or singing, or dancing!)

Are You Ready for Gusto?

Learning to like yourself is one of the most important steps you can take on your road to health. You do not have to accept living a life in which you are uncomfortable with yourself, your body, and your health. You are a work in progress. Change is often the hardest challenge we face in life, but you must not be afraid to face it. Most of us have gotten pretty used to the way we live. We want to change, but we're uncertain how to replace those old habits.

Something sparked inside of you that made you go to the bookstore and lay down your hard-earned dollars to buy this book. Could it be you *might* be *ready* for a change? Making room in your life for something new is always a positive step. It'll keep you creative and motivated. Part of the wonder of being on my program is that with each and every step you take, you challenge a different facet of who you are. Because this is not a "diet" program, but a Total Health Makeover, you get the opportunity to get to know yourself from the inside out. Spend time looking at your face, your body (all sides of it) in the mirror. Study the pieces of the puzzle that make the whole of you. Acknowledge what you see and accept the flaws. (We all have them, that's for sure!)

What happens too often is that we become so discouraged with the distance between where we are and where we want to be that we give up the fight. We make excuses for why we "can't" change the way things are. Maybe you're too old, too set in your ways, or just too embarrassed to put on a leotard, let alone allow anyone else to see you looking so out of shape. The idea behind gusto is to break those self-imposed barriers. Guess what? An old dog *can* learn new tricks! Put on that tutu and dance around your house. Break that sweat every day. Build your confidence as you build your health. You must silence that pessimistic voice of self-harassment in your head (that ugly mirror) that holds you back. Becoming aware of that voice is the first step in quieting it down and finally making it go away. If you start to have negative thoughts, so what? We all have them! Have *all* your feelings. Your feelings are not going to kill you. Just use judgment when putting your feelings into action. And remember, accepting who you are and all of your feelings that come with it, is gusto!

My "Toy Box" Theory

I have a theory that everyone has a little drama they deal with in life. I call it the "toy box" of feelings. We create a box of little dramas and problems to keep us busy enough to avoid the real major issues that are holding us back. To avoid becoming the person you want to be, or achieving your goals, you take out this little toy box and you play with your problems. For me, it was always those last five or ten pounds. It's funny that being thirty-five or forty pounds overweight didn't bother me as much as those last few pounds. (Especially because I am an actress, a career in which you are judged by your looks more often than your talent.) I always avoided dealing with some other drama in my life because it was easier for me to play with my "weight" toy. I kept blaming my excess weight for not getting some part in a movie or television show. I knew how to diet and I knew all about food. It was always so convenient for me to play with those toys instead of dealing with the real issues that were holding me back either in relationships or in my career. In 1981, I finally looked the way I wanted to look. I was at my ideal weight. And you know what? I still wasn't at a place in my career where I was satisfied! I didn't have a valid excuse anymore, because the weight toy was put away. I had lost those ten pounds I had always blamed for my other misgivings. I realized that the weight wasn't the problem but a manifestation of my other issues. In a panic, I re-created that problem as a safety zone. I was comfortable being a little up in my weight because that was easier for me to confront. I called those extra pounds my body armor. They protected me from the outside world . . . or so I thought. This type of behavior is easy to see in all areas of your life. Maybe you always pick the wrong partner or wrong job. (I had a history of picking guys that were impossible to have a relationship with.) Once I realized what I was doing, I came to the conclusion that life is a cycle of circles. During 1981–1987, I allowed my weight to go up and down and up and down. I was in a bad marriage, I was nervous about my career after *Taxi*, and my weight just started to creep back on. But I learned that this was self-defeating behavior. Once I made up my mind that I could be my worst critic *and* my own best friend, I got strong, made the decision to live a balanced life, and haven't looked back since. The nice thing about a toy box is that you can keep the toys you like, play with them when you feel like it, and put them away when you're done.

Looking Good, Feeling Good

We all want to look good and feel better about ourselves. Self-improvement isn't just about aesthetics. "You" are not your body. "You" live *within* your body, and it's important to make that distinction. There are so many areas of your life you can be proud of, but it all stems from within. The pressure placed on us by society to look thin, youthful, and sexy are all driving forces behind this desire to base your attitude on how good or bad you look. There's no other book that will say this to you, but I will! It *does* matter how you look as long as *you* feel it matters. When I was up in my weight, I was unhappy with the way I looked most of the time; no one else knew it, but it bothered me. And even with all my gusto, there was always some part of me holding back. It's funny . . . I went through hundreds of old pictures while making my selection for this project. My friends helping me cracked up because in every photo, no matter how awful I looked, I had such attitude! The first photo session where everything came together was with famed photographer Harry Langdon. I had been on my program for two solid years, and was finally in the condition I had hoped for all my life. I really wanted to be in shape for the shoot. This was the first time I had my hair, makeup, and wardrobe professionally done for a photo session. (I wore thirteen different outfits!) After twelve hours of shooting, I was exhausted and exhilarated. When I saw the pictures, I couldn't believe it was me. This was a fantasy come true to do a photo shoot like this. But even more important, it was a dream come true because I really looked like my idealized image of myself. For the first time ever, what I was feeling on the inside was captured on the outside. As shallow as it sounds, and as much as we hate to admit it, it does matter how you look and what you put out there to other people. If it doesn't, then why is everyone's projection of self tied to appearance? There are tons of studies that show looks matter when searching for a job, a date, and even friends. However, if it doesn't matter to you (be honest), then God bless you!

But even if you aren't where you quite want to be physically, you can get through any situation with gusto. I remember appearing on *The Tonight Show* when Joan Rivers was the guest host. I felt really fat that day but couldn't back out of the appearance. I said to myself, "Please God, she can ask me my age, or how I lost my virginity, but please don't let her ask me how much I weigh!" I secretly hoped I'd come down with the flu, but I didn't and I made that appearance. I carried myself with gusto (or fake gusto, AKA gusto zirconium) and had a great time that night (although she *did* ask me how I lost my virginity)! Ironically, my husband, Rob, whom I didn't meet until six months later, saw the show that night and swears he fell in love with me from that appearance. Sometimes faking *is* better.

> *"Too much of a good thing can be wonderful."*
>
> MAE WEST

You'll always have something that you'll want to change about yourself, because as long as you live and breathe, you will remain a work in progress. The ultimate reward in improving yourself is that you will inevitably improve your health and your self-image.

As with the rest of my program, once you take that first step to attaining gusto and putting faith in a positive attitude, you can't help but graduate to another layer because the changes you're making for yourself are working. You'll start to realize that people are noticing the "new" you. Maybe it'll be a compliment from your boss on how good you look. Perhaps your tennis partner will notice you're hitting the ball a little harder than usual. You're not afraid to lock eyes with that handsome stranger across the room. You're walking taller, with your shoulders back and your chest out. There's a lightness that surrounds you. You breathe easier, your senses are sharper, and somehow you have become more aware of your surroundings. You're no longer afraid to look yourself in the eye (let alone anyone else).

Are you wondering, "How do I get there?"

Confidence and Self-Esteem

Change your thoughts and you change your world.
NORMAN VINCENT PEALE

You know the saying, "Be your own best friend"? It probably stems from the fact that we are undoubtedly our own worst critics. It's incredible how a few wrinkles or extra couple of pounds can shatter the way people view themselves. Self-esteem and self-worth hit an all-time low at the discovery of a "happy birthday" flaw. (I always feel like after my birthday I receive some gift from the God of Aging.) Developing your confidence and self-esteem can have tremendous positive results in your Total Health Makeover. Someone who possesses genuine gusto is likely to respect her body and will eat better, get enough exercise, and avoid wearing herself down both physically and mentally. Someone who is self-assured doesn't feel angst over the small stuff in life. She doesn't create scenarios that don't exist. Molehills hardly ever become mountains. Confidence gives you the courage to seek and to try new things, and to constantly challenge the world in which you live. Find something you love to do and then become *your* best (not *the* best) at it. Pursue something that really excites you, and go for it with gusto. Don't fear failure, because it is really just an opportunity for setting your sights on a new success. Think about it this way. You've been on a zillion diets, and with each and every one you've had some success and some failure. Remember that even if you strive for something and never quite reach your original goal, you will always gain some unexpected knowledge, insights, and rewards because of your quest. Life is a trial-and-error process, and you won't grow unless you try, and sometimes that means failing in that attempt. Beating yourself up emotionally for failure does a lot more harm to your psyche (confidence and self-esteem) than the actual failure does.

As you become more confident and self-assured, there's a snowball effect. The more confident you become, the more confident you become. I know it seems so obvious, but it's so true! It's part of that winning syndrome mode. It's a regular two-for-one special!

Gusto and Food

One of the main principles behind this book is that something goes in, something gets processed, something comes out. Nothing that goes in will get processed successfully unless the energy flow is uninhibited. So what does this mean to us? Let's say you're going out for a BIG dinner with a bunch of friends to your favorite restaurant and you're planning to eat anything and everything—in other words, you're going for "numb" tonight. The worst thing you can do is to sit there saying, "Oh my gosh, I shouldn't be eating this, I'm off my diet, and I'm going to hate myself tomorrow." I'm telling you that no way is anything in that stressed-out body going to get digested. Every cell in your body will horde from the stress of that negative energy. However, you should say, "Hey, I am out for a good time tonight, I'll make up for it tomorrow (by properly food combining, or jumping on that treadmill, or drinking a lot of water) but tonight LET THE GOOD TIMES ROLLLLLL!"

If you obey all the rules you miss all the fun.
KATHARINE HEPBURN

Setting Goals—A Road Map to Gusto

Set goals for yourself. Each time you accomplish a meaningful task, you feel really good about yourself, don't you? It's the same theory here. Goals are an essential part of life. They give us hope and something to reach for. Meeting those goals fills us with great pride, vitality, and boundless energy.

Setting goals keeps you moving in a forward direction and adds a great sense of worth to your well-being and purpose. Without having something positive to go for in life, we become weak and unfocused.

Literally write down your goals on a piece of paper. This act makes you feel more committed and your goals become tangible. Make this list a virtual checklist and mark off each goal as you reach it. Once you make the list, prioritize which goals are most important for you. Concentrate on the things that you are seeking when you make that list as opposed to the things you don't want. That keeps the tone positive. Set a deadline so you know how long you have to meet the challenge. Give yourself a break if you don't meet that deadline. You didn't fail as long as you are on the way to meeting the goal. A deadline simply gives you something to aim for. Make sure you update your goals and keep adding new ones as you meet them along the way. Circumstances change, and what seemed important to you six months ago might not be a priority today. The psychological challenge of setting and achieving a goal is to your mind what exercise and healthy eating are to your body.

Imagery and Visualization

Imagine that you had the ability to see your future, and that you can hit the fast-forward button in the VCR of your mind to see yourself six months from now. What do you see? (Close your eyes for a moment and try this.) Are you thinner, richer, happier? Imagery and visualization are a therapeutic process in which mental pictures play a central role in helping the mind influence the body. If you can think it, you can be it. The centuries-old (it's been around since the thirteenth century) technique is predicated on the idea that our minds can influence the unseen processes of our bodies. Imagery and visualization rely on the assumption that there is a direct and powerful link between the mind and body. Before I shoot a movie, go on stage, or appear on a talk show, I always try to get a clear mental image of what my appearance will be like. I get a vivid picture of how I want to look and how I want to behave, and the strong image of success I want to achieve, in each of those goals. Imagination and memories can be used to mentally smell, taste, see, and hear images that you are trying to achieve. As an actress, I've been trained to exercise each of my senses to create a moment in a character's life. I use this training to do my homework and help create a realized moment in my own life.

> *The mind is its own place, and in itself can make heaven or hell . . .*
> JOHN MILTON

If you can imagine yourself healthy, vibrant, successful, a winner, you can be all those things by adding a little gusto to your life.

A footnote to the story about my friend Cynthia . . . one year after that romantic weekend, I was named godmother to the beautiful little girl born from that union.

Talk about working the coat!

14 | Why Certain Diets Work and Others Don't

Die-it

I thought about renaming this book *Die-it? or Live-it!* because that is what I truly think of when I think of dieting. The act of depriving your body of food and its essential vitamins and nutrients goes against the basic laws of nature. To purposely put yourself in a state of starvation is to die a slow death. Why on earth would anyone knowingly do that to herself? When I started on my journey to fitness and health, I had a lot of trial and error along the way. I had to find a way to keep moving in a forward motion regarding my health. In the past my diet ritual was one step forward and one step back. Sometimes it was two steps forward and three steps back. What I eventually discovered was that my experimentation led me to a new cycle, one that propelled me in that forward direction I was so eagerly seeking. Eventually, the pattern became two steps forward, and one step back, until ultimately there was consistent forward motion with occasional (hey, I'm human) small steps back. The one thing that I discovered with absolute certainty is: *YOU MUST EAT REAL FOOD TO LOSE WEIGHT AND BEGIN A HEALTHIER LIFE.* That's right, you heard me correctly. You *must* eat real food (not fake, chemical-laden powders, drinks, or food) to lose weight.

A recent George Washington University study shows that the leanest 30 percent of the American population eats the most amount of food. They are also the most active and healthy group of the population. How much you eat and exactly what you eat makes all the difference in whether you will win the battle against your weight. Our bodies need carbohydrates, protein, and fat to survive. If you deprive yourself of any one of these, you will be out of balance. The food we eat has a huge effect on how we think, feel, and act. Simply reducing calories won't necessarily result in weight loss. The body is an extremely functional machine when treated properly. In the simplest terms, I've always had this mental image of little men inside our bodies shoveling coal into a big hot furnace. If they run out of coal to keep the fire burning, the stove just shuts down. Putting fewer calories in your body won't solve the problem because your body is meant to work at its maximum. If you don't feed it properly it cannot run as efficiently as it should. You've got to give those little guys the coal to keep the fire burning. If the body isn't sure where its next calories are coming from, it views any sudden drop in caloric intake or energy supply as a threat. The body readjusts itself to adapt to that change, and learns to get by on very little coal (or calories). That's why when people go on a very low-calorie diet for a period of time, they will lose weight. But as soon as they go back to their regular eating habits, they will put the weight back on (and then some), because the body has set itself up for the famine. That's why we need eating habits that we can live with every day, as opposed to a "diet" that is not intended for long-term use.

I have seen every diet fad come and go and come around again over the years, and what I have discovered (especially after trying every one of those fads) is that there is no substitute for eating a "balanced" diet (as discussed in Chapter 2) that you can live with. There are some quick fixes, but surely you know by now that you cannot sustain weight loss and live a happy normal life on those programs. Hey, I admit it. I have gone on "crash" diets in the past to get in perfect shape for some event. Who hasn't? I'm not saying that once in a while you can't go that route, but I am suggesting that the *need* to need that in your life can be and will be greatly diminished by changing your relationship to food once and for all. And that's the true essence of what this book is all about. It's not a program of deprivation, starvation, or some wacky "Hollywood" fad diet. It's an honest-to-goodness organic way to live your life. It is doable, it is attainable, and above all, it is long-term. Make the choice to start on this program today, and step by step you will get to a place where this program is as normal as brushing your teeth, and it will be as natural as breathing in and out all day long.

> *Eating a diet based on grains, vegetables, fruits, and beans can save a family of four around $40 per week or $2,100 a year. You could buy a new car after six years.*

Don't confuse this book as another fast way to achieve your weight goal. It is not a quick fix. Most diet programs are about a feast or famine mind-set.

FEAST——— FAMINE

You are usually at one extreme or the other if you're a typical yo-yo dieter. It's simply an unnatural relationship to food. This up-and-down approach only makes you feel worse in the long run because it doesn't teach you how to live as you should. Somehow I figured out that I would never have to live a life of famine again if I could reconcile the feast and strike a balance. What I'm showing you is how to live in the middle of these two extremes.

Live-it

Feast—————Marilu's Program—————Famine
Feast—————B.E.S.T. Program—————Famine

My overall idea is not only to show you how to lose weight, but to teach you how to be a healthier version of yourself. You can be thin and unhealthy, and likewise heavy and healthy. I know a lot of people who would fit each of these descriptions. I want to help you change your approach and relationship to food and eating. Making that connection is the best way I can think of to keep you on this path to health. I always knew that I had to discover a program that I could live with every day and not feel deprived. I wanted to eat foods that I liked and to teach myself how to really taste the food I was eating. The results were dramatic and comfortable. The more I discovered that this was leading me toward feeling the way I wanted to feel, the more I wanted to prolong the effects.

It has taken a lot of fine tuning and acceptance to realize that even on those days where I might not follow this program exactly as I should, it is in no way a failure. I'm human and so are you, and there will be those days for sure. Just knowing that you can do something to counterbalance the indulgence should help you confirm that this is a lifestyle program and not just another diet.

I think women today are not as interested in their health as they are in their weight and jeans size. Thin is in, right? WRONG! Health is in. In fact, if asked, most men would prefer a women who has an athletic body over the stick-thin waiflike models thrust in our faces on the covers of all those fashion magazines. As women, we tend to be harder on ourselves (and each other) and try to conform to our own expectations of what we think we should look like. We're motivated by our own standards, and that's fine as long as the goals are realistic and fall into a healthy, reasonable look.

Diet Roulette

According to the American Medical Association, 30 percent of all adult Americans are overweight. The reason so few dieters win the war against their weight is that most are victims of their own body. They have successfully messed up their metabolism over a period of years, and they simply can't figure out how to undo the damage. There is a simple explanation to maintaining your weight.

In theory, the calories consumed must equal the calories you burn. So logic tells you that reducing your caloric intake should equal weight loss, right? Well, sorry to tell you, not exactly. A lot of variables impact individual results. Factors such as genetics, metabolism, emotional state, physical activity, and of course eating habits (the types of foods you're eating, the quality, timing, and the combinations) are just some of the elements that can affect your ability to lose weight. So what do you do? There's a ton of conflicting information out there, and no wonder. Even the experts can't agree on what is the best approach to weight loss. The only two things they can agree on are that regular exercise is important and that obesity is unhealthy. But there's so much more I have learned about weight loss and health.

> *Close to 50 million Americans are dieting right now, and most will not lose the weight they want.*

Some critics say that your chance of sustaining long-term weight loss with a diet is about the same as winning the lottery. The Institute of Medicine claims that despite the billions of dollars spent each year on weight loss, very few people will reduce their weight to their desired level, and even fewer will maintain that weight loss. Well, guess what this is telling us, folks: DIETS DO NOT WORK!

With all the programs available to you, how can you know which is the safest, most effective one to choose? Weight Watchers,

Jenny Craig, Optifast or SlimFast, diet pills (over-the-counter brands like Dexatrim and the controversial prescriptions like Redux and Phen-Fen), and the list goes on and on. It's truly a game of diet roulette, and in the end you may be the one who gets the bullet. Dieting and weight loss, like most industries, is a money-making machine. Every person I know who wants to lose weight is willing to spend hard-earned dollars on it. There has never been any convincing truth that

> *The annual cost of obesity in America is $100 billion, which includes the $33 billion Americans will spend on weight-loss products and programs.*

short-term weight loss will result in improved long-term health for the average overweight dieter. In fact, the weight usually returns, and that in itself can be more detrimental to your health than being overweight. Most dieters are choosing programs that promote quick weight loss and not a lifestyle change. Most of those programs never address the bigger issues of how a dieter relates to food or how to be healthy or how to maintain a normal existence while eating in a restaurant. Eating a "candy bar" (like those diet bars) for

> *Ninety-five percent of all dieters will fail at their attempt to lose weight.*

lunch is not going to cut it as a way of life. Maintaining the rigidity of these programs is impossible for most people. But most importantly, factoring in all the other aspects that can affect your results is extremely important to better your odds in this game of roulette.

A Mayo Clinic study of several hundred obese patients showed that one-third of the patients were overeating, one-third were eating normally, and the last third had low metabolic rates. That's why it is incredibly important to discover a program, like I did, that balances out all the perils and pitfalls of short-term weight loss and a long-term lifestyle change.

Men Versus Women

Here's a little fact for you. More adult women are considered clinically obese than adult men, but by only a small margin—34 percent women and 31 percent men. Oddly enough, more women are, by a far greater margin (50 percent) trying to lose weight than men (25 percent). Society puts an enormous amount of pressure on people,

> Men burn an average of fifty more calories an hour than women do.

especially women, to be thin. We've all seen those talk shows that exploit the discrimination against obese people. We have seen the humiliation that those people suffer because they can't fit in an airplane seat or get a job because of their appearance. Women in particular push themselves to achieve the cultural ideal picture of being thin, often to the point of being harmful and unhealthy. I knew a woman in dance class who had starved herself to such a degree that her body actually started growing furlike hair all over her body as a defense mechanism to keep warm. Her body just couldn't offer up that circulatory function anymore because she was vitamin- and nutrient-starved, so in its survival mentality, her hormone levels changed, causing the unwanted, albeit needed excess hair growth to protect itself.

When weight loss is strictly for aesthetic reasons, ultimately you doom yourself for failure. The up-five-pounds, down-ten-pounds, up-twelve-pounds cycle only leads to total frustration. This constant frustration, of course, just adds to the vicious cycle.

Childhood Eating Habits

I believe that society puts an inordinate amount of pressure on women to look a certain way, starting as early as childhood. It's no mistake that books such as *Reviving Ophelia* have been on the bestseller lists for months and months. It is a book that deals with teenage weight loss and the mentality that young girls develop because of societal expectations and through watching their own mothers' behavior. It all starts at home, and how your children are taught to approach food and their eating habits. Not too long ago, I was teaching my son Nicky all about the importance of eating protein. I explained to him that protein will help him grow big and strong. Nicky asked me if his favorite dancer, Michael "Lord of the Dance" Flatley, ate protein, and I assured him that he did because he needs to keep lean and strong as a professional dancer. The next thing I know, Nicky had his head in our refrigerator and I asked him what he was up to. With great determination, he said, "I'm looking for soybeans, Mommy, so I can have some protein right now!"

Kids can be taught to eat healthy or unhealthy. It's up to us as parents to set the example and explain the difference. It's really hilarious when Nicky has a friend over for a play date and the mother comes to pick up her son and can't believe I could get her kid to eat veggie burgers or soy cheese pizza when all he'll eat at home is macaroni and cheese. His friends leave asking their moms to make them a snack like Nicky's because it looks better and tastes better, too. Kids are smart, and they'll eat good-tasting food, even if it's healthy.

Overeating is a learned behavior and a trained response. If you were sick as a child, your mother probably fed you. Feeling a bit sad? Try eating your troubles away. Trends for obesity in children in America virtually mirror the adult statistics. An estimated 27 percent of American children are overweight. Kids have become far too sedentary today. They would rather sit at home in front of their computer playing video games, or watch television than play outside with their friends. This inactivity has greatly affected the obesity rate among children. It starts young sometimes because children observe their parents' attitudes about their own bodies. (I know a little girl who didn't want to wear a dress to her third birthday party, because she didn't want to show her "fat thighs.") Experts agree that children under the age of ten should not be put on a diet, yet in a recent *Nutrition News* study, a group of ordinary-weight ten-year-old girls were surveyed, and all of them said they would feel better about themselves if they were thinner.

Childhood is when your eating habits are developed and influenced the most. Parents have maximum control over what a child eats and how a child will view food. If a child is brought up in a household with bad eating habits, the likelihood of that child continuing those habits into adult life is almost certain. If children are taught to "diet" at an early age, more than likely they will spend the rest of their lives struggling with their weight and their relationship to food. The struggle will be even more difficult if during one of two key stages of life they are severely overweight—either as a baby or during puberty.

Once children reach their teenage years, they discover that what they eat is basically the one thing they have absolute total control over in their lives. That epiphany results in the alarmingly rising rate of bulimia and anorexia among teenage girls and the rapid weight gain some adolescents will experience when they leave home for the first time. You may recall the term "freshman ten" for first-year college students who gain ten pounds their freshman year at college. A 1987 survey of high school students found that 63 percent of all the girls surveyed were dieting as opposed to 16 percent of the boys. Virtually all the obese girls were dieting, as were 66 percent of the average-weight girls and 18 percent of underweight girls. Only 50 percent of the obese boys were dieting and 25 percent of the average-weight boys were dieting. These are pretty startling statistics, and certainly a commentary on our society and the pressure we all are faced with regarding our appearance.

> *Eighty percent of the people suffering from anorexia and bulimia are women.*

Overweight Men and Women

In the days of the caveman, it was believed that men needed more muscle because they were the hunters and gatherers of food.

Women needed a higher fat-to-muscle ratio because they were the baby makers and needed to keep their young warm and protected. Researchers agree that being overweight can be a greater health risk to men than to women. Men are likely to carry excess weight above their waists in their bellies, which is strongly associated with heart disease, Type II diabetes, and other health-related ailments. Women are far more likely to seek medical attention for their weight problems than men, and again, it is probably due to societal pressure placed on women to look a certain way. A Cogan and Rothblum study shows that overweight men and women are less likely to get married. Overweight women are less likely to be accepted to elite colleges, tend to earn less money, and are more likely to be poor than normal-weight women. All this leads me to ask a very important question here. Is it the excess weight that holds back these people, or is it society and our judgments that overweight men and women can't possibly function as well as normal-weight men and women that holds them back? It would seem that societal oppression is a far greater problem than being overweight, though being overweight certainly presents its health risks to the individual. If the media would stop placing such an emphasis on the supposed desired look a man or woman *should* have and focus on teaching a *healthy* approach to eating and losing weight, we would all be better off.

When I first started to look at the principles of weight loss, it was almost as if I were given a certain number of cards to play with every day, and once I used them up, I was done for the day. Well, guess what? I realized that there were cards in that deck that I wasn't even meant to have! I discovered that I wasn't meant to eat dairy products (I'm not a young calf). And because I don't have all canine teeth (only four incisors that are meant to break open grain), meat is something I'm not supposed to be eating either. I didn't need those dairy and meat cards anymore. My greatest revelation in learning how to eat healthy once and for all was learning exactly what my body is capable of breaking down and using most efficiently. Weight loss is not meant to be just about aesthetics, but about overall health and well-being. It's a reprogramming of the way you think about and approach food. Women and men need to feel better about themselves and not just better about their outward appearance. If you eat well, there's no way your health and appearance aren't going to change for the better.

The No-Fat Explosion

When I think of fat, I always get an image of old film footage where women would put themselves in these machines that vibrated and shook their fat wherever the belt was placed on their bodies. It's like an old episode of *I Love Lucy* that keeps flashing through my mind. The only way to get rid of fat is to reduce your fat intake, but there is no such thing as a "fat-free" diet. You're kidding yourself if you think that you can possibly survive without some fat intake. Of course, you could try living only on foods that contain little if any amounts of fat, like vegetables and fruits, but how boring is that? Eventually, you will starve your body of protein and carbohydrates and those old cravings will kick in. Our bodies need fat, but somehow we have gotten to a place in this day and age where everything we eat is now "fat-free." Well, fat-free doesn't exactly translate to healthy or low-cal. In fact, nutritionist Richard Mattes conducted a study on how people alter their eating habits when they think they're eating a fat-free meal. He found that when people were given meals that had the same fat content as their usual meals, but were told that the fat content was lower, they ate more. They ate so much more that even if the food had been lower in fat, they would have consumed more fat than usual. Mattes believes that this is what happens with adults who are going nuts buying up all those fat-free cookies, chips, and other foods. The biggest problem as I see it is that people eat senselessly. I find that most people don't think about what they're putting in their mouths, and are eating excessive amounts of empty calories. Not to mention all the chemicals the food manufacturers have to add to their fat-free products to make them taste edible.

Fat in food is what makes it taste so good. Flavor adheres to fat, so that explains why all the "fat-free" foods on the market today have very little (if any) flavor. Our palates have gotten so used to the flavors of food laden with heart-clogging, artery-thickening fat that we can't taste the simple flavors in food anymore. That's why the "fat-free" food companies have to add so many chemicals to their foods, so we can *taste* something. If you removed the fat without replacing the flavor, the enormously successful fat-free and low-fat food business would quickly become a total bust.

When dietitians convinced people to get off fat, they didn't anticipate the increase in carbohydrate consumption, which can turn into fat if eaten to excess. One gram of fat equals nine calories. One gram of protein or carbohydrates equals four calories. When you eat fat it is used either to lubricate or to heat the body. Any excess fat gets stored as fat, because it doesn't have to go through a chemical change to become fat. On the contrary, *excess* proteins or carbohydrates make a chemical change within the body, which turns 25 percent (meaning 75 percent of the calories get used in the process) of the intake into fat. In the simplest terms, even though excess fat is nine times more fattening than excess proteins or carbohydrates, you still end up loading

> *Ninety percent of all Americans now buy reduced-fat, low-fat, or no-fat foods.*

up on more proteins and/or carbohydrates than your body needs or can use when you eat only fat-free foods. That is the best explanation as to why almost everyone who went on a fat-free eating spree didn't necessarily lose weight.

Nutritionists literally okayed it for us to eat more protein and carbs because they had fewer calories. Though the government recommends a diet that derives 30 percent of its calories from fat, a recent National Center for Health Statistics study showed that most Americans are well above that amount at around 37 percent, and that most health experts (and I) would prefer a 25 percent level to achieve true healthy eating.

The absurdity that people complain of gaining weight while eating a so-called low-fat diet typifies the American approach to food and losing weight. As a society, it seems we'll do almost anything to lose weight, except what it really takes: *balancing our diet with the foods we are meant to eat!*

Is There a Magic Pill?

NO.

Okay, so maybe I ought to elaborate a little bit on this topic since it has certainly been newsworthy over the past few years. We can take a pill to battle disease in our bodies, prevent unwanted pregnancies, and eliminate muscle aches and pains. In this immediate-gratification society we live in, it makes sense that people are looking to solve their weight problem by taking a diet pill or appetite suppressant. In severe cases of obesity only, prescription medication *may be* helpful in helping that person to shed pounds. Research shows that appetite suppressant medications, *when combined* with changes in diet and physical activity, can help *some* obese patients lose more weight than those not on a drug-therapy program. Taking these types of medications can help sustain weight loss, and in general they are safe only when used under the care of a physician. They are not recommended for long-term use or for patients under 30% overweight. But don't confuse taking these drugs with the answer to permanent weight loss, because like any other diet method, the drugs do not teach you to readdress your approach to food. There is a false sense of being satiated when taking these drugs, because most trigger a chemical response in the brain that falsely tells your body that you are full. The drugs affect neurotransmitters in the brain, such as serotonin, which play a role in altering your mood. As soon as you stop taking the medication, you'll be right back to your old eating habits. Anyone who thinks that she can go on these drugs for a short period of time, lose the weight, and then go back to her old eating habits is setting herself up for weight gain and that vicious cycle all over again. Another type of drug awaiting FDA approval is Orlistat (Olestra), a fat blocker. It helps block the absorption of fat in the intestine. The side effect is anal leakage, diarrhea, and other intestinal disorders. Another issue with taking a medication to lose weight is that there has been a long history of addiction and misuse of these products, which can bring about tremendous side effects, such as heart problems, respiratory problems, and dependency. To date, every diet drug ever devised for weight loss has been mass-marketed before it has been proven safe and effective. Phen-Fen and its recent recall off the market is a perfect example of pharmaceutical companies attempting to cash in on Americans' desire to cure their weight problems with a magic pill. At what cost? Your health! In the laws of nature, anything that is unnatural, like taking a pill, has some sort of payback or drawback. That is the ebb and flow of life. Your weight gain was not a quick and easy process, so it stands to reason that your weight loss will not be, either.

What Is Obese?

Most of us don't have a very accurate body image when we look in the mirror. Knowing whether you are a candidate to lose weight becomes very subjective. "Obese" is clinically defined as being 20 percent or more above the normal weight given for your particular age, height, and frame size. Obesity rates around the world vary because of eating habits. Researchers say that 60 percent of obesity cases can be traced to some genetic flaw in countries where the food supply is abundant, meaning that there is such a thing as a fat gene, but that is not an excuse for being overweight or obese for most people. Overeating is an unnatural eating pattern. Your body wasn't meant to consume the massive amounts of food most people ingest on a daily basis. Of course, eating habits are affected by all sorts of factors, both external and internal. An internal impulse may be the sound of your stomach gurgling to let you know it's hungry, or you may feel a dip in your energy level, which is a signal that your blood-sugar level has dropped. External stimuli might be the smell of something baking or a buffet that looks delicious. It might even be something as simple as a regular eating time, like a set lunch break from work. Your body clock goes on autopilot and knows it's time for lunch before you can even look at the clock. These are all pretty normal eating responses. What happens to people with a compulsive eating disorder is that they will eat whether they're hungry or not. They have very little if any control over their appetite and food consumption.

One in three Americans is seriously overweight. Obesity is now considered an epidemic in this country. Obesity can lead to heart disease, cancer (especially breast cancer), high blood pressure, high cholesterol, immune problems, gallstones, diabetes, arthritis, stroke, and sleep apnea. Various explanations can be given to explain why people are fat, but the one that stands out as making the most sense is that most overweight people eat too much of the *wrong* foods. I don't want to sound insensitive, because I know it's not easy, but the truth is, it's that simple. I know, because I've been there. I eat more food now than I ever have. I'm eating the right types of food and properly food combining. Body type and genetic predisposition contribute to this fat epidemic, but you can take steps to avoid the external learned behavior that is keeping you overweight.

To change your eating behavior is to modify your relationship with food, and you control that 100 percent by virtue of what you put in your mouth. Without getting too deep here, unhealthy eating habits are often a disguise for a much larger problem in your life. Overeating will always make you feel lousy, but eating to escape from whatever else is making you feel crummy is not a problem solver. Eating for comfort is an unwise choice. The real formula for weight loss and weight control is to eat a centered diet, avoid extreme foods, avoid unnatural foods, exercise, and do not overeat.

Finding Your Ideal Weight

Standardized tests are a horrible way to test individuals. Unfortunately, they're all we've got to work with, so they are used for almost everything. I have the same feeling about weight charts. My suggestion is that your ideal weight is within a certain range of weight. Any woman can tell you that her weight can fluctuate as much as five to ten pounds for a number of reasons. Lack of sleep, drinking alcohol, PMS, flying, and, of course, diet issues such as excessive salt, which causes water retention. I say your ideal weight should be based on what feels good to you and what is healthy. Use how your clothes are fitting as a barometer. If I gain weight, I gain it like a man, around my midsection. If I have to unbutton my jeans to sit comfortably, I know that something is out of balance in my routine. (Too many late-night dinners, not enough exercise, etc.) Conversely, I know that if I fall below a certain weight, my face looks too drawn and emaciated and it's not as attractive. (Catherine Deneuve once said that after thirty you go for your face or your butt!)

Get to know your body and the reactions you have to food and eating patterns. You have to *get* in touch with how you feel in order to *know* how you feel.

Readjusting Your Weight Set Point

One of the things I noticed when I was getting in touch with my body is that I would go through periods that no matter what I did, the scale weight would stay the same. I didn't realize that there was actually a name for it at the time, but I later found a magazine article that defined this phenomenon as your "set point." In general, you can diet and lose a few pounds, but have you noticed that your weight most likely creeps back toward that old familiar spot on the scale? Our bodies tend to defend a certain weight, which is the weight your body tends to hover around, not unlike hitting a dieting plateau. Your set point isn't an exact number but more like a range of numbers that your weight tends to fluctuate between. Your set point is actually a result of the combination of the size and number of your fat cells, your resting metabolic rate, and other factors such as exercise and eating habits. You can readjust your set point by permanently changing your eating habits and modifying your exercise program. I finally readjusted my set point (by fourteen pounds!) by adding twenty minutes of aerobic activity every day. That was the final element that I needed to break that plateau and be my B.E.S.T.!

With so much conflicting information out there and the mega-choices you have for diet programs, it's no wonder most people fail at their attempt to lose weight. Who could effectively diet in such a state of confusion? It's enough to want to make you just run out and grab a bacon double cheeseburger and a milk shake. While I won't directly bash any specific diet, I will say that most programs don't work for long-term weight loss and weight management.

15 | Is Heredity Destiny? To See Your Future, You Must Know Your Past

*H*aving lost both my parents at a fairly young age (and both from potentially preventable diseases) I realized that tracing your family health history could be the most important step you will ever take toward living a healthier, longer life. Knowing your roots and learning your family health history will help you identify any genetic or predisposed health inheritances and will help you avoid these perils if possible. Any disease that runs in your family puts you at risk. Once you discover the health problems various family members have had, you can figure out how these can affect you and what you can do to protect yourself from getting these conditions. Inside each of us is a genetic blueprint that is passed on from each generation. It contains a plan that dictates our future. I knew that I'd possibly been dealt a heart attack and arthritis card from my family deck, so I made damn sure that whatever cells I built up in my body and the food that I ate were able to help combat those diseases.

Sometimes we stumble into our future and sometimes we create it.
ROGER SMITH, FORMER PRESIDENT OF GENERAL MOTORS

Is Heredity Destiny?

Your chances of inheriting health defects are high. Ignoring family illnesses guarantees their place in your future and the future of generations to come. Identifying those red flags early can save lives, and not just yours, but also the lives of other family members. A child born to parents who are both insulin-dependent diabetics runs a one in ten chance of inheriting diabetes. The risk can be greatly diminished if that child exercises regularly and maintains a healthy weight. Children of alcoholics are approximately three times more likely to become alcoholics. If you recognize a pattern of alcoholism in your family, you can seek help to avoid becoming an alcoholic yourself. The idea is to look for that red flag. If you are aware of what to look for you can take positive action in preventive medicine for your own health. You can also make your doctor aware of signs to look for. That's why most doctors ask about family history on your first office visit. It helps them guide you to seek the healthiest road and to know all your options.

The best way to know your family history is to seek out all the proper information and record it. I've developed a Family Health History Chart to help you gather all the information you'll need. Look for patterns and common ailments from both sides of your family. Cancer, high blood pressure, heart disease, diabetes, depression, arthritis, and even alcoholism are all common and potentially life-threatening diseases that you can do something about. Try to find out at what age your family member developed any of these diseases. If a family member died of heart disease in his eighties it's not as big a concern as a family member developing heart disease at age thirty-five. Although doctors agree that there is some genetic component to any disease, don't make yourself crazy if you find a pattern. It does not mean that you will automatically develop that disease or condition. In fact, knowing about the likelihood of occurrence greatly helps diminish your chances of affliction. In other words, having a diabetic grandfather raises your risk of diabetes, but it does not necessarily doom you to the disease if you make the necessary changes in your lifestyle.

Likewise, a clean record does not mean you have nothing to worry about, and you can just whoop it up and let yourself go. There are silent conditions that may have gone undetected in the past that may be hovering somewhere in your future. High blood pressure and high cholesterol are two such conditions. So it's important to get regular checkups and follow a healthy program.

An ideal family health history includes details on all your close relatives, both living and dead. Collecting the data can become a daunting and time-consuming task, but make it a priority. (And make it fun . . . you never know what you might uncover about your crazy old relatives!) It may someday truly save your life. I know that some of you would rather not seek out this type of information for fear of what you may find, but I urge you to gather it, because knowledge is a good thing even if the news is bad.

Don't stick your head in the sand, because it's *never* too late unless you wait too long! Ignorance is not bliss. In this case, it's just plain stupid.

Your first focus should be on older family members, since they've probably already shown signs of certain diseases that are in your bloodline. You'll want to get information on your grandparents, parents, aunts, uncles, and all your siblings to complete a thorough health history. If you're married, do the same gathering of information for your spouse and your spouse's family. This is especially important information for your children, even before they're born. Before I had my first son, Nicky, I had amniocentesis at seventeen weeks. The doctors wanted to know everything about my spouse and me, so I ended up filling out quite an extensive family history questionnaire for the test. I now have a better understanding of our past and our son's future.

The following list will help you gather pertinent information for each of your relatives. The goal is to gather as much of this information as possible. Learning as much as you can about your family history is as close as you will get to having some control over your destiny. Remember, *knowledge is power!*

As you question relatives, you may feel like you're uncovering family gossip, but on the other hand, you may learn that there have been some diseases that are not genetically linked to your family, because someone you considered a relative has no "blood" relation to you, such as a stepparent, an adoptive family, or a relative through marriage. (Okay, so maybe you might be gathering a little family gossip here, but again, knowledge is power.) This is the information you need.

* Full name and date of birth for each family member.

* Complete marriage history, including divorce and remarriage information.

* Height and weight of each family member.

* Average amount that each family member smoked and drank alcoholic beverages.

* Any health problems, including chronic headaches, frequent colds, allergies, birth defects, and even broken bones.

* Occurrences of heart attacks, strokes, cancers, asthma, diabetes, high blood pressure, high cholesterol, miscarriages, and all major surgeries.

* Age at the onset of these conditions.

* Any cases of depression or substance abuse, including suicide attempts.

* Date and cause of death for each family member. Be thorough about the actual cause of death. For example, if a family member died of cancer, what *kind* of cancer did he have?

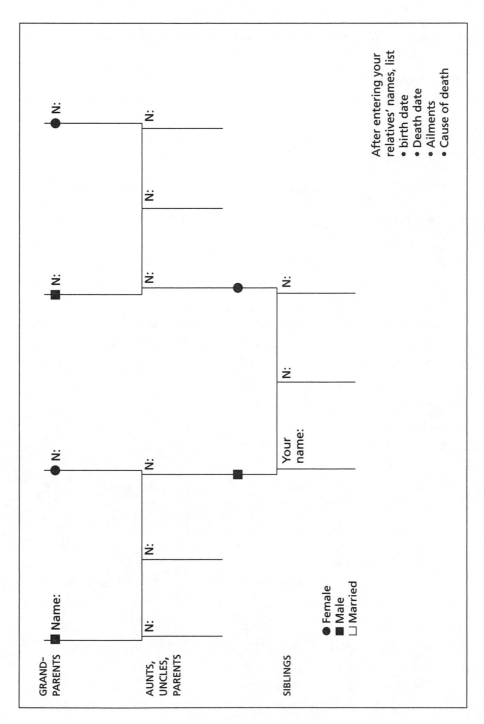

GRAND-
PARENTS

Name:

N:

N:

N:

AUNTS,
UNCLES,
PARENTS

N:

N:

N:

N:

N:

SIBLINGS

Your
name:

N:

N:

After entering your
relatives' names, list
• birth date
• Death date
• Ailments
• Cause of death

● Female
■ Male
☐ Married

189

Understanding Your Genes

I've got my mom's eyes, my dad's nose, and I inherited the ability to rumba from both of them. Does this mean that I might have arthritis or suffer from a heart attack like my parents? It may have, but I'm taking control of my life and fighting back by eating healthy and taking care of my body. More than 4,000 disorders have been found to result from defects in single genes. Many other ail-

> *The life of a human cell ranges from one day (a cell lining the intestine) to ten years (a white blood cell).*

ments are triggered by the interaction between several genes and outside factors. But as I said earlier, disposition does not mean development. Chronic illnesses like heart disease and diabetes tend to be caused by an interaction of genes with environmental factors, such as diet and physical activity. Heredity doesn't mean certainty, but it can if you don't take the proper precautions now. Even if a disease is known to run in your family, where and when it might strike is the great unknown. So you may want to consider genetic testing to help prove whatever your family health history suggests. We all walk around with defective genes, and our ability to detect the ones that aren't working is far greater today than ever before. You want to make sure those

> *We have between 50,000 and 100,000 genes in our body. There are 75 trillion cells in our body. If you counted one cell per second, it would take over 2 million years to count them all.*

genes don't get their chance to mutate and take over. You can stack the deck in your favor if you know what to look for.

Therefore, every day of your life you have the choice to make better and more improved cells for your body by consciously improving the quality of your life, *or*, by continuing an unhealthy lifestyle, you can choose to continue to make defective and less vibrant cells, which will eventually break down, making you more susceptible to disease.

I've outlined a list of common genetically inherited diseases. In each and every case, you can take precautions to prevent or at least diminish your odds of inheriting the disease.

Obesity

Defined as being 20 percent or more over your ideal body weight, obesity can increase your risk of heart disease, hypertension, and diabetes. Obesity afflicts one in three adults in America and one in four children. Obesity is not linked to any one single gene, but genetic factors are possible. There are known "fat genes," and you should be conscious of other family members that have constantly battled the bulge. Patterns of growth can be inherited, and genetics can contribute to how fat you are and your body shape, but it's not mandatory, so don't use heredity as your only excuse. Obesity can also be and often is caused by environmental factors such as eating habits you learn from your family. You can control obesity by following a healthy and well-designed eating program and doing regular aerobic exercise. Exercise speeds up your metabolism and will help you shed the weight. There's no great revelation here, because these are the facts. But I'm here to show you that hereditary obesity doesn't have to be your destiny.

High Blood Pressure

Often called the silent killer, high blood pressure can lead to heart disease or a stroke. High blood pressure is easy to detect and easy to control. If one of your parents has or had high blood pressure, you are 25–50 percent more likely to develop it. If you had a parent who handled stressful situations by getting "red in the face" and always seemed to be on the verge of exploding, you may want to check for that behavior in yourself. Stress management (finding a better way to deal with things) might be a good idea. In addition, most people with high blood pressure have high-sodium diets, which raises your blood pressure, so the number one prevention on the list is to cut salt (especially table salt) from your diet. Eating potassium-rich foods, like bananas and potatoes, also helps keep the blood pressure down. As with obesity, exercising regularly and eating a healthy diet are surefire ways to improve your blood pressure.

Heart Disease

Because heart disease was a particular concern of mine, I was especially interested in the facts, and what I discovered was staggering. We now know that heart disease is the leading cause of death in women. Almost half of all heart attacks happen to women, and nearly 9 million women die each year from heart disease. Heart disease kills twice as many women as *all* cancers combined. This is a serious concern, and many genetic factors such as blood pressure, cholesterol levels, and weight affect your likelihood of suffering from some sort of heart disease in your lifetime. Having a parent with heart disease raises your risk of having heart disease. The younger the parent was when the illness developed, the more likely you are to develop some form of heart disease. Again, environmental factors must also be considered, like smoking, eating a high-fat diet, and living a sedentary lifestyle. The good news is that the effects of almost every risk factor can be turned around. The obvious first step is to *eat a low-fat, dairy-free diet*. This will help lower your risk almost immediately. *Don't smoke*. Some experts think smoking is the number one factor that causes heart disease. *Keep an eye on your blood pressure*. High blood pressure puts a lot of unnecessary pressure on your arteries, which overworks and weakens your heart. You can reduce your risk of a heart attack 2–3 percent for every point you reduce your blood pressure. *Staying fit* is once again a key factor in keeping your heart healthy. Women who are even moderately overweight are 80 percent more likely to suffer from heart disease. *Stress management* is important because stress can also trigger heart disease. A Harvard study claims that 40 percent of all heart attacks occurred within two hours after a psychologically stressful event. Another recent study that followed 100 men over a thirty-year period found that those who were angry more often were three times as likely to suffer a heart attack and nearly six times more likely to suffer a stroke at mid-life. So try to reduce your stress level to help the fight against heart disease.

Depression

One of the least talked about secrets is that almost every family has at least one person who is emotionally derailed and/or suffers from depression. Crippling sadness, noticeable weight gain or loss, the need for excess sleep or insomnia, can all be symptoms of depression if they last more than two weeks. If either of your parents has suffered from depression, you are more likely to develop it than someone whose parents do not have this condition.

Being moody should not be confused with being depressed. Clinical depression is actually a genetic flaw in the brain's chemical fight-or-flight system. Clinical depression is an illness, but the symptoms are behavioral rather than physical. Depression can be triggered by a traumatic event that really makes someone feel helpless. Losing your job, losing a loved one, the breakup of a marriage or relationship are all common adult traumas that can bring on the darkness of depression. Two major factors will determine just how deep into the abyss you fall: your genes and your childhood. According to Frederick K. Goodwin, M.D., former director of the National Institute of Mental Health in Bethesda, Maryland, and now the director of the Center on Neuroscience Behavior and Society at George Washington University, "Genetic vulnerability is the single biggest predictor of who will get clinically depressed and who is not. The brain mechanisms that go awry in depression are the ones programmed by the brain to control the so-called fight-or-flight reaction." So in someone who is genetically predisposed to depression, once an event triggers that response, there's no turning back. Proper counseling can help you work through this stressful time, and should shorten the length of your depression.

The other predictor of depression is your childhood. Events such as abuse, the death of a parent, or even a case of being bullied at school can directly affect how you handle stress and depression today as an adult. Conversely, being overindulged and overprotected shields a child from the realities of life, and that in itself can manifest symptoms of depression later in life for an adult who is trying to cope. Obviously I can't go into depth on this subject (that would be a book in itself), but if you suspect that something from your childhood is affecting your life as an adult and might be partly responsible for your depression, seek counseling.

As many as 61 percent of all people diagnosed with depression may actually be suffering from other diseases in addition to their depression. Depression might be a side effect of prescription drugs you are taking. Some 5–10 percent of women who take oral contraceptives also find that depression is a common side effect, caused by the synthetic hormones used in some pills. Some 10–15 percent of people who are depressed have a thyroid imbalance. Here's one you might recognize . . . people who get depressed in the winter. It's a real disorder, referred to as Seasonal Affective Disorder (SAD), which is caused by not enough sunlight. Many women show signs of depression before (PMS) or during their periods, or during menopause. Certain symptoms can be alleviated by avoiding extreme foods (anything too salty or too sweet) and alcoholic beverages, and adding a few extra complex carbohydrates to your diet during these times. These foods, as well as increased physical activity (taking a walk, playing tennis, even dancing around the house), will help boost serotonin levels in the brain, which will help stabilize your moods.

The best defense against depression is to recognize its symptoms and get help.

Cancer

It seems to me that cancer is such a twentieth-century disease. Maybe it's that we're constantly hearing on the nightly news about something else that is giving lab rats (let alone people) cancer. We're bombarded with the threat of cancer all the time. Years ago (and not that many years ago), people whispered in hushed tones about the Big "C" almost as if it were a curse from God, not connected to anything else. Of course, we now realize that cancer is virtually surrounding our every move. Aside from hereditary propensities, cancer can be caused by environmental factors, the sun, food additives, radiation, polluted water, asbestos—the list goes on and on.

One in eight women will develop breast cancer, and 5–10 percent of these breast cancer cases are inherited. Researchers have identified at least two genes linked to this disease. Some 10–15 percent of all cases of colon cancer are inherited, and 20,000 new cases each year are directly related to family genes. Cervical cancer, skin cancer, lung cancer, even ovarian cancer, all have these same types of startling statistics. Likewise, all these cancers can be greatly diminished if you take the proper precautions to avoid the perils of such diseases. If you look at these statistics and think that the percentages are relatively small, think about what that is really saying. The other causes of these diseases must be linked in some way to your eating habits or other lifestyle choices, over which you have control. That is the essence of my message throughout the pages of this book. If you don't fit into the stats here, the cause of any cancer you might develop may be directly related to these other factors, and you can and should be doing something to improve your health. And if you *do* fit into these statistics, you had better decide *now* that there is something you can do to lower your risk.

Osteoporosis

Your bones are the steel frames for your body. They are supposed to be the support for all your internal organs and act as a structure upon which you can depend. What happens to those (women in particular, because osteoporosis strikes four women for every man) who start to lose their strength and skeletal structure because of the onset of osteoporosis? Osteoporosis is a steady, progressive loss of bone density that causes bones to become fragile and brittle. It will strike one in every four women. If afflicted, you become prone to easily fracturing a hip, your spine may become hunched, and you will be at risk for all sorts of other bone-related injuries. You will not only look older as a result of osteoporosis, you're going to feel older, too. Because of the sensitivity of your bones and skeleton, you'll become far more cautious about participating in any activity that might put you in jeopardy. Osteoporosis can be prevented if you take the right steps toward correcting the already decaying skeletal structure in your body.

Women have less bone than men to start with, so this crippling disease is particularly dangerous for women. It can really have a devastating effect after the onset of menopause. Because there's a drop in estrogen during menopause (this helps hold calcium in the bones), osteoporosis often occurs when a woman is "going through the change." Postmenopausal women will lose 2–3 percent of their bone density per year and will continue to lose it at that rate for the first five years after menopause. Osteoporosis can strike at any time, however, and if your bones are thinning before menopause, you will definitely need to replace the calcium in your body by taking supplements or starting hormone therapy. If you don't tend to the problem it will develop into a serious case of osteoporosis. Severe cases can result in shattered spines, severe back pain, and the "incredible shrinking woman" syndrome (meaning you'll actually get shorter!).

An estimated 25 million Americans suffer from osteoporosis.

To know whether you're at risk of developing osteoporosis, you need to understand your family history of this disease. If your mother had osteoporosis, you would be considered a 50 percent greater risk candidate. Up to 70 percent of your peak bone mass is determined by heredity. Petite women have a higher propensity to the disease because they have less bone mass than larger-boned women. Bones get stronger and tend to build during the teenage years and continue to build through your thirties. You develop two types of cells during this time. If your bones are getting stronger, the osteoblasts (the bone-building cells) are outgrowing the osteoclasts (the bone-destroying cells). Your bones will reach their optimum level of strength in your thirties. From then on, it is a battle (although one you can successfully win) to keep your bones strong and healthy.

Women who eat a low-calcium diet are at a greater risk of developing the disease. Calcium is one of the essential minerals needed to build strong bones. The National Institutes of Health recommend that premenopausal women get 1,000 milligrams of calcium per day, though many experts think it should be even more (around 1,200 milligrams per day). Menopausal and post-menopausal women need at least 1,500 milligrams of calcium every day to keep their bones nice and strong. (Look at the Calcium Rich Food Chart on pages 89–91.)

As with every disease I have mentioned so far, exercise is a key component to warding off the onset. Leading a sedentary lifestyle just makes you a lethargic, unhealthy, unhappy blob. Exercise stimulates bone growth, and without it, your bones can become more fragile. Smoking and heavy drinking can also have a negative effect. Smoking in particular is believed to drain the levels of estrogen from your system, making it more difficult for your bones to absorb what they need to stay strong.

If you think you're a candidate for osteoporosis, there are steps you can take *now* to strengthen your skeleton and keep "dem bones" healthy.

* *Calcium* is to your bones what gasoline is to your car, or blood to your heart. Without it, you can't function. You need calcium to stay healthy. Some 99 percent of the calcium you

ingest goes straight to your bones. Without it, you can't replenish lost bone matter. Although most people think that dairy is the best source for calcium, it is in fact a poor source. (See chapter on Dairy.) Green leafy vegetables, salmon, nuts, tofu, and beans (such as garbanzos and pinto) are all excellent sources of calcium. Citrus foods also tend to leach calcium from your bones, so limit your intake of citrus foods as well.

* *Vitamin D* is helpful in fighting the onset of osteoporosis. Bones can't absorb calcium unless they have enough vitamin D. Without it, your body absorbs only 10 percent of what it would absorb with enough vitamin D. Vitamin D helps the small intestine prepare for the oncoming accumulation of calcium. You can consume vitamin D by eating certain foods, like bread and cereal, or you can take an oral vitamin supplement.

* *Exercise*, especially weight-bearing exercise, helps stimulate bone growth. Exercising at least three times a week for at least twenty to thirty minutes is ideal. Focus on strengthening your lower extremities (your back and hips). The bones that are most vulnerable to injury as a result of osteoporosis are the hips and the spine. Walking, running, swimming, and aerobics are all good ways to strengthen those extremities.

Osteoporosis does not have to affect your life if you take proper precautions to avoid the perils at an early age. Most of the information I am providing in this book will help you prevent or at least lessen the odds of contracting any of these diseases, especially ones you might be genetically predisposed to developing as you age.

Diabetes

Most people probably think diabetes is a disease you're born with, but the truth is that most people develop this potentially serious disease between the ages of thirty and forty-five. More than 14 million Americans have diabetes, and approximately 5–10 percent of them are insulin-dependent. Diabetes occurs when there are abnormalities in the body's production or use of insulin. As a result, blood sugar can rise to a high level, and in severe cases cause blindness, kidney failure, or heart disease. If you are an adult living a sedentary lifestyle (cleaning the house is the most exercise you get, and that's on a good day!), you are a prime candidate for Type II diabetes. Type II diabetes can have less severe

> *A woman with diabetes is six times more likely to have a heart attack than a woman who does not have diabetes. She is twenty times more likely to suffer kidney failure, and five times more likely to suffer a stroke.*

symptoms, such as blurred vision, frequent urination, unusually high thirst, or cuts and bruises that seem to take longer to heal than usual. The warnings of this type of diabetes are often so vague that many people who suffer from it don't realize it until it's too late.

As you can see, it's so important to know your family history to help you avoid potential bouts with any of these (and other) diseases. Once you know what you can do to keep yourself healthy, you'll be better able to stay healthy. Understanding all of this information is a useful key for your entire family, so I really encourage you to seek all of the information you can to be prepared. There's no way of predicting a completely disease-free life, but you can do something to curtail your chances if you know how.

16 | Reading Your Face

I filled in for my good pal Kathie Lee Gifford as guest host on *Live with Regis & Kathie Lee* in December 1997, and the wildest thing happened. I was chatting with Regis Philbin about my book, during the "host chat" segment, and he asked me what was going to be so different about this book. He was sort of teasing me and suggesting that a health book is a health book is a health book. (But by now, you know that this is no ordinary health book!) Well, to tell you the truth, I don't think Regis was quite ready for my response. I told him that I was going to include a chapter on how to "read your face." Reading *his* face wasn't that difficult after my announcement. He was clearly shocked, if not stunned. I, of course, was thrilled. (It's not often Regis is speechless.) I challenged him to ask me more questions about explaining the telltale signs that are *all over* your face if you know how to read them (a pimple in a certain spot, or puffiness in a certain area). I explained that these manifestations are usually an indication that something is "out of balance." Michael Gelman (the show's executive producer, and the cutest guy) was offstage pointing to the pimple on his chin he had gotten recently. When I told him that it was probably from too much salt, he admitted, "I love salt. I ate a whole bag of potato chips this weekend!"

I felt vindicated, and better yet, the audience wanted to know more.

Many years ago I discovered the practice of "Oriental Diagnosis," and I had experimented with it on friends and myself and now I finally have the chance to share it with everyone through this book. There is so much we can interpret about what's going on in our bodies through this ancient medicinal practice.

According to Michio Kushi, the author of *Oriental Diagnosis— What Your Face Reveals*, "The standard Oriental writings on the causes of disease stressed the relationship between an individual's health and his or her diet, activity, spiritual attitude and total environment. No single aspect of human life was considered separate from another." This sounds so obvious now, but nineteen years ago, when I first read these words, this belief was not the norm. Long before I was born, and until fairly recently, traditional Western doctors (including my childhood pediatrician) made their diagnoses based solely on observing already existing symptoms. It was rare for a Western doctor to consider the whole picture, including family history, diet, and environmental factors. But Oriental diagnosis foresees the development of a disease before any symptoms are visible. (Today, I take my boys to a pediatrician who balances these two schools of thought.)

Your face, eyes, hair, and skin are some of the best indicators of what's happening with your health. Have you ever noticed a pattern of breaking out from stress? How about a zit that pops up in the same place over and over again? Maybe on your chin, forehead, or cheek? Have you ever observed that people who smoke have puffiness around both sides of their noses? Guess what . . . this is telling you something!

How to Read Your Face

Your face can be divided into three sections, each coordinating to a different system in your body. Your forehead region from the eyebrows and up correlates to your nervous system. This is the yin section of your face, and if you eat too many yin foods, like candy, sugar, tropical fruits, and alcohol, you'll show the signs (redness, pimples, and a rash) in this region. Your mouth and chin region below the nose corresponds with your digestive system. This is the yang section of your face, which is affected when you eat overly yang foods, like excessive salt, beef, animal fats, and processed foods like lunch meats. The third region, which is the rest of your face including your cheeks and jowls, has to do with your circulatory system. Smokers, heavy dairy eaters, and people who are going through hormonal changes are prone to breakouts or puffiness in this region.

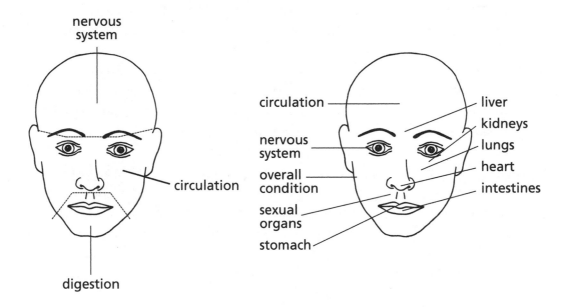

Each of these regions can be further divided into more specific areas that correspond to an organ or body function. For example, if the tip of your nose is red or swollen, it *could* indicate a genetic predisposition to a heart condition. Swelling or deep circles under the eyes could be a sign that your kidneys aren't functioning properly or are being overtaxed. Puffiness on either side of the nose could be a warning of a bronchial problem or indicate that your lungs are clogged from too much smoking or overeating dairy products.

Heavy vertical wrinkles above your nose and between your eyes could indicate a problem with your liver. You might want to watch your consumption of excessive yang food and/or alcohol. Heavy horizontal wrinkles on your forehead could indicate a problem with your circulation. You might want to watch your consumption of excess liquids, especially drinks with chemicals and/or alcohol. The area above the upper lip corresponds to the sexual organs. If there is a horizontal wrinkle in this area when you smile, there could be a weakness in the sexual organs. Such a wrinkle in men could indicate weak sexual vitality. In women, it could mean a menstruation problem. This wrinkle is often associated with eating too many animal products, including all dairy products. (Another great reason to get off dairy!) Vertical lines in the area above the upper lip could mean that the sexual organs are shrinking. (This is another great reason to give up smoking, which can create these lines and constrict your veins—everywhere.) Maybe this is why so many guys grow mustaches!

The different parts of the lips correspond to your stomach. The top part of the lip is connected with the top part of your stomach. The middle part of the lips correspond to the middle part of your stomach, and the lower lip section corresponds to the lower stomach. The lower parts of the corners of your mouth are connected to the gall bladder, liver, and pancreas. The mid-part of the lower lip can indicate a condition in the intestines.

I know, I know. Right now you're saying to yourself, "What the heck is she talking about?" When I first read about this it sounded a little bit "out there" for me, too, but it really seems to work! Whenever I get a pimple on a certain part of my face, it *always* relates to the "right" wrong food. I can't tell you how many times people have asked me to read their faces, and when I've spotted a certain weakness, and call someone on it, I usually get a look of surprise and sometimes denial (especially when I nail a closet smoker). But please . . . your face doesn't lie. And don't get freaked out if you have a little puffiness here and there. It doesn't necessarily mean you have a heart condition or are dying of lung cancer. There's no reason to overreact. It can simply mean that compared to your other organs, one particular organ may not be as strong or that you may have a genetic predisposition to a sensitivity in that organ. Look at the illustrations on page 202 and try to read your own face by using these as a guide.

Getting Under Your Skin

Genetics, behavior patterns, environment, and diet are all major factors in how your skin ages. Your skin goes through major changes as you mature. With each decade from your twenties on, you have to pay special attention to what your skin goes through on a daily basis. When we were teenagers, a pimple could make our hormonal world crash and burn at the first hint of a bump. Believe me, I know. At age fourteen I was called "Braille face" because of all the little pimples on my forehead. Little did I know it was because of all the candy I consumed every day. When I outgrew candy and moved on to more adult food, like gourmet cheeses, my cheeks broke out as well. I can't tell you how many doctors have told members of my family, "It's not what you're eating that's causing the breakouts." It's funny though, as soon as we gave up certain foods, our complexions cleared up. A myriad of factors can affect your skin in many different ways. If you know what to be wary of and take proper care of your health, you will grant yourself the gift of aging gracefully. Some changes in the face are inevitable with time. The severity of those changes can be avoided.

As we get older, the fat layer that lies beneath the skin and contours the face thins out. The skin produces less collagen, which is the spongy protein that gives skin its bounce. The stretchy fiber in the skin (elastin) gets weak, so the skin doesn't snap back like it used to after being stretched. That's why your skin loses its snug fit as you age. Your complexion changes as you age, too. It becomes dull-looking and dry. The new cells at the bottom of the epidermis (your outer layer of skin) take longer to reach and replace the cells on the surface of your skin. What took your cells two weeks to accomplish in your twenties takes a month by age fifty. The dead cells give your skin that uneven look, which is why you might notice a flaking of your skin you never had when you were younger.

> *Nature gives you the face you have when you are twenty. Life shapes the face you have at thirty.*
>
> COCO CHANEL

Wouldn't you know that it was the fabulous Coco herself who launched the sunbathing craze in the 1920s? She returned from a cruise with a deep dark tan, and single-handedly turned the tan into the fashion "must have" for the decade. Of course, by now we all know what kind of damage the sun can do to our skin, including early aging, not to mention skin cancer. I was never one to sit in the sun. Even as a kid I didn't like being in the sun too long, because a sunburn was so uncomfortable. Unfortunately, many people will have the rest of their lives to wear the damage innocently done. Those of you who avoided exposing your skin to the wrath of the sun will have significantly different-looking skin than those who baked their faces. The sun is just one factor that must be considered when you analyze your face and skin. To some degree, you can reverse the damage to your skin caused by overexposure to the sun. Staying out of the sun and wearing sunscreen when you are outdoors will allow your body time to rejuvenate and increase its collagen level, which makes skin suppler. You won't turn back the hands of time, but you will have healthier-looking skin.

Ninety percent of the lines, wrinkles, and blemishes on the face are not caused by aging, but by toxins (including those found in food) polluting our system. From age thirty and on, 5 percent of Americans will suffer from adult acne, which can cause red skin; spider veins around the cheeks, nose, and chin; and breakouts. People who blush easily and have fair skin are the most likely candidates.

Fair skin is very thin and is prone to freckling, age spots, blotchiness, and broken capillaries. Darker skin tones like olive or brown skin are blessed with a natural tendency not to wrinkle. The drawback here is that darker skin tones can look leathery and weathered if the skin is damaged. These skin tones have more melanin (the natural chemical in skin that allows it to tan) in their genetic makeup, so they are less prone to wrinkles but can still look weathered.

Besides eating well and staying out of the sun, the one-two combination of exfoliating and moisturizing is another great way to care for your skin (especially in winter weather). Exfoliating removes the top layer of dead skin cells. Moisturizing helps keep the healthy new cells moist. This causes them to swell and cluster, giving your skin a smoother, less-wrinkled appearance.

> *An estimated 17 million women in their twenties, thirties, and forties struggle with adult acne.*

Pollutants outside and inside the body can build up in the skin and cause a dry, damaged-looking complexion. A moisturizing face mask can help free the trapped toxins and leave your skin looking radiant, healthy, and rejuvenated. While everyone knows that you can take care of your face, surprisingly enough, the lips are often an ignored, yet important part of the way we look (and kiss . . .). You might have perfect skin but your lips could look like the surface of a dry desert. Exfoliating your lips sloughs off dead cells from the surface, eliminating lines and cracks, and leaves your lips looking healthy and younger-looking. Special lip exfoliants are designed to help remove the dry and loose skin from weather-damaged, dehydrated lips. (I particularly like the lip exfoliant sold at The Body Shop.) You should also try drinking more water (the hydrating cure-all) to avoid chapped lips.

Stress is a catalyst in more than half the cases of adult acne. Outbreaks are most likely to occur two days after the onset of some emotional struggle. (I'm sure that your circulation, digestion, and nervous system are all affected.) Although dermatologists have long maintained that stress affects skin, only recently has strong scientific evidence emerged showing exactly how this happens. Researchers at the University of Pennsylvania School of Medicine have found a protein called Substance P that is secreted by nerve fibers in our organs during heightened anxiety. It may cause the skin's tiny blood vessels to become clogged with white blood cells, resulting in inflammation. One's emotional state can play a large part in skin irritations. In fact, some researchers believe that the excess of sweat produced as a result of stress causes breakouts because it clogs the pores on the skin's surface. Reducing the amount of stress (or learning how to handle it in a better way) can improve your complexion in the same way changing your diet does. Dermatologists are being trained these days to look for extenuating conditions before writing a prescription. Years ago, doctors offered only topical solutions, which included dry ice treatments, antibiotic creams, sulfur salves, and cortisone shots. Today, they're looking for "solutions" beneath the surface of the skin. It stands to reason that if you balance things on the inside, they're likely to become balanced on the outside.

Vitamins and Minerals That Help Your Complexion

Your body converts beta-carotene into vitamin A, so eating a healthy dose of beta-carotene every day helps generate new skin cells and protects your skin against skin cancer. Apricots, peaches, nectarines, sweet potatoes, tomatoes, spinach, and carrots are all great sources of beta-carotene. Vitamin C is essential in building new collagen. Citrus fruits, berries, melon, tomatoes, papaya, spinach, and sweet potatoes are good sources of vitamin C. Selenium, another antioxidant, found in fish, garlic, chicken, and grains, works with vitamin E against pollutants, sunburn, and skin cancer. Selenium helps maintain the quality of the skin. It functions internally to help close wounds. You can find selenium in protein foods; tuna, shrimp, and poultry are good natural sources of this healing mineral. Since vitamin E is hard to get from food without eating too much fat, the best sources are oil-rich nuts, seeds, and avocados. Calcium is important for preventing sagging skin and wrinkles. The best calcium sources are broccoli, spinach, tofu, salmon, and soy products. (See Chapter 8 for more calcium-rich foods.)

The average cost of a facelift is $4,000. Surgically removing bags under your eyes costs around $2,200. A forehead lift costs $2,000, and the cost to get rid of a double chin averages $1,300, depending on the size.

Well, if that doesn't put this chapter in perspective for you, nothing will. Hey, this book cost only $15! I'd call that money well spent. So many people spend their hard-earned cash to get the fat sucked out of their cheeks, chins, and under their eyes, when maybe what they *should* be doing is giving up smoking, dairy, meat, and sugar.

17 | What's the Poop?

*P*eople say you can divide the world into two groups. Some say it's leaders and followers. Others say *Tonight Show* versus *Late Show* fans. And still others insist it's those who pay retail and those who pay wholesale. *I* say you can indeed divide the world into two groups. There are those who can openly discuss bowel movements and those who find it unthinkable. I, of course, fall into the first category and feel it is my duty (make that doody) to bring this usually malodorous subject to your attention. I will boldly go where no author has gone before. I want to make your "business" my business. It's funny that people easily talk about the most intimate aspects of their lives, and yet somehow the subject of evacuation and bowel movements (a very normal part of our human existence), makes some people squeamish and uncomfortable. Well, I'm here to finally remove that stigma from your life and make bathroom talk okay for any room. Hey, it's a dirty job, but somebody has to do it! While I recognize that this chapter might come under all unrelated "doodies," it's high time a book tackled this topic and put to rest any and all fallacies about feces. We have put men on the moon and found cures for the rarest of diseases, yet with the possible exception of predicting the weather, no topic is so prone to uninformed information.

Have you ever wondered about the origin of the saying, "What's the poop?" Why in the world would that question somehow be translated in modern-day English to mean "What's new with you?" or "Tell me what's going on in your life"? Clearly, someone along the way, perhaps a wise philosopher, knew something important that has been passed down from generation to generation. Perhaps the idea is, if you know your poop, all other knowledge shall follow.

It is best when the stools are soft and formed and passed at an hour customary to the patient when in health.

HIPPOCRATES

Your Digestive System and How It Works

To understand what "normal" bowel habits are, you must first have a general understanding of your digestive system and how it works. This might sound a little clinical, but look at the digestive chart and follow the path food and liquids take on the journey of digestion. Remember, it's not the destination that counts, it's the journey, right?

> *Over the course of seventy years, the intestines process forty tons of food, at about one inch per minute.*

The digestive system is a series of hollow organs joined in a long twisting tube from your mouth to your anus. Inside the tube is a lining called mucosa. In your mouth, stomach, and small intestine, the mucosa contains tiny glands that produce juices to help digest the food you eat. Digestion happens when food is mixed and moved through your digestive tract and is chemically

210

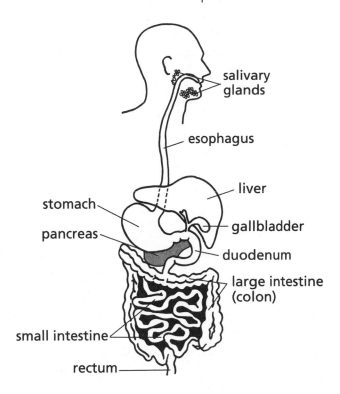

salivary glands

esophagus

liver

stomach

gallbladder

pancreas

duodenum

large intestine (colon)

small intestine

rectum

broken down from food into smaller molecules. Imagine that your colon is a long tube with small hairlike fingers (cilia) along the sides. These "fingers" pull nutrients from the digesting food, sorting and sending the nutrients to where they need to go in the body. The remaining undigested fiber gets passed further along through your digestive tract.

Digestion begins in your mouth as soon as you start to chew, and your brain sends a signal to your stomach that the food is on its way. It's really important to thoroughly chew your food because *your stomach doesn't have teeth.* (Unchewed food could flatten the cilia along the walls of your colon thereby inhibiting the nutrients from being "pulled" through the system.) Digestion is then completed in your small intestine. When food or liquid is first swallowed, it is initially a voluntary choice, but once swallowing begins it becomes involuntary and is actually controlled by nerves. (Envision yourself gulping down a glass of water and think about that *glug, glug, glug* sound.) The swallowed food is pushed into the esophagus, which connects the throat with the stomach. Once the food enters the stomach, it goes through three different stages. First, the stomach must store the swallowed food or liquid. This requires the muscle of the upper part of the stomach to relax and accept large amounts of swallowed material. Remember those signals sent to the stomach by the brain when the food was first eaten? The second job is to mix up the food and liquid with digestive juices produced by the stomach. These are mixed together by the muscle action in the lower part of the stomach. The third task is to slowly empty the contents from the stomach into the small intestine. Several factors can affect the emptying process of the stomach, including the nature of the food (mainly its fat and protein content) and the degree of the muscle action of the emptying stomach and the next organ to receive its contents. As your food is digested in the small intestine and is dissolved into juices from the pancreas, liver, and intestine, the contents are mixed and pushed forward to allow further digestion. The final stage of digestion occurs when the nutrients are absorbed through the intestinal walls. The waste products (the stuff we don't use) of this process, including undigested parts of the food, known as fibers, and older cells that have been shed from the mucosa, are propelled into the colon. They remain for about a day or two (or longer if you're not healthy), until the feces are expelled by a bowel movement. And that, my friend, is truly the poop!

Whew! I'm so glad I got that out of my system.

> The human body has about twenty feet of small intestine and six feet of large intestine. The total surface area is more than 100 square feet, which is five times the area of your body's skin.

The Poop on Poop

Now that you have a brief understanding of your digestive system, it's time to get a little up close and personal. How well do you know your poop? Do you have any idea what your bowel movements really mean?

Frequency of Elimination

The average American (around 97 percent) has from three bowel movements per day to three per week. This seems a bit wide in range, but if you fall in this range, you are considered "normal" according to a 1982 study by Drossman and others. There may be day-to-day variation in frequency, but most of you will still fall well within this range. (However, if you are eating the B.E.S.T. way, you will be going at least once a day.) Several circumstances can affect your bowel movement habits. You may be aware of factors such as traveling and eating different foods you're not used to, but did you know, for example, that women often find a change in their movements during their period? Heat can encourage more bowel movements, while cold conditions may inhibit them. Marathon runners have a higher frequency of diarrhea. You might say they get the runs . . . (sorry, but I had to . . .). If you do not fall within this "normal" range, you should see a doctor immediately. If you're not sure how often you actually make a bowel movement, keep a diarrhea . . . I mean diary. Put a little note pad and pen in your bathroom at home and keep track for a few weeks. You should be able to identify your pattern within three to four weeks. I know this sounds a little offbeat, but one of the best barometers of how our body is functioning is an understanding of what comes out of it. Maybe that's why it's become a compliment when someone says you really "know your shit."

Hey, we talk about it for babies, we talk about it for older people, why is all the time between those stages the lost years?

Stool Weight

Have you ever gone to the bathroom and immediately jumped on the scale after making number two? (I'm a mom, remember?) I know you thought you must have lost an easy two-three pounds by the looks of it. Well, I hate to break the news to you, but the average stool weight is 4.2 ounces. A lot of factors besides the food you're eating can affect the actual weight of your stool. Malabsorption of fat results in bulky, softer stools. Failure of the small intestine to absorb fluid and electrolytes may produce a larger stool. Dietary fiber can increase stool weight because fiber absorbs more water.

> *An outgoing personality or a positive self-image may be responsible for more stool weight.*

I love this fact because it demonstrates to me that someone who is easygoing and doesn't hold on to a lot of tension is going to have an easier time with normal bodily functions.

To tell you the truth, there is very little reason to know the actual weight of your stool, but sometimes it can help a doctor determine if there is a problem. In general, your poop should float. This is always a shock to people, because most people pass "sinkers." You want "floaters," as I like to call them. That is what you have to look forward to when assessing the healthiness of your stool. Nothing gives me greater pleasure than to have a new devotee to my program joyously announce her breakthrough of seeing her poop float for the first time. Lillie Kae Stevens, one of my castmates in *Chicago* and a Marilu convert, recently burst into my dressing room with overwhelming pride. She had just passed her first floaters since starting my program, and boy was she excited. This may be more information than you need, but life *is* about sharing our happiest moments, right?

Floating poop is an indication that the food you're eating is properly balanced, not too contractive and not too expansive. If it's hard and sinks you've probably eaten too much protein. If it has a sheen and leaves skid marks, too much sugar. I'm not saying that every time you go to the bathroom you'll have perfectly colon-shaped floaters, but it is a great gauge for what's going on in your body.

Transit Time

Transit time is the length of time it takes for food to move through your body. The shorter the transit time, the less chance you have of the food becoming toxic in your body. It takes around eight hours for the food to travel through the stomach and small intestine. The rest of the time it spends in your body is spent in your colon. A person who's eating a healthy diet should pass that food within twenty-four to forty-eight hours.

As your body starts to work more efficiently, the transit time should be within twenty-four hours. Don't expect to be in this range immediately because your body needs to readjust itself to your new healthy ways.

Stool Consistency

The value in understanding the consistency of your stool lies in understanding the difference between being constipated, being "normal," and having diarrhea. There is actually a tool called a penetrometer that measures the distance traveled into the stool of an average poop dropped from standard height. Fortunately, this device is not commonly used, so don't worry about your next trip to the gastroenterologist. Interestingly, a stool that appears well-formed in the toilet bowl might actually be soft and mushy if it were to fall to a hard surface, so judging consistency is not a consistent science. In fact, it's a pretty subjective observation. For our purposes, the following standards are used to describe constipation and diarrhea. Constipation is hard, dry, and sometimes painful to pass stool. It can also be described by an infrequent urge to go. Diarrhea is loose, watery stools. An increase in regular movements may also describe elements of diarrhea. Anything between these two extremes is usually called "normal" bowel movements. We're going for optimum health here, so your goal is eventually to go daily like clockwork. The stool should be colon-shaped and pass with relative ease. Small foods, such as corn that hasn't been properly chewed, do not process well in our system. Have you ever wondered why corn, for example, appears whole in your toilet, even though you swear you chewed it going down? Now you know why. You're probably not chewing your food enough. If lettuce or larger foods are coming out whole and undigested, this can be a sign that you're not chewing your food properly as well.

Effort

How much effort you make when evacuating your bowels is really important. In fact, the force generated, the time required to pass the stool, and even your position on the toilet are important factors to consider to establish a normal pattern. If you strain more than 75 percent of the time, you probably suffer from regular constipation. On the contrary, loose, watery stools more than 75 percent of the time probably means you suffer chronic diarrhea. Straining can actually be hazardous to your health. It can pop hernias, distend hemorrhoidal veins, and even cause gastric contents to reflux into the esophagus. It's funny if you think about it. We're the only animals on earth that need reading materials to go to the bathroom. Is it going to be a *People* magazine or a *War and Peace* kind of poop? And you never ever see animals in the woods making groaning sounds when they have to go. Of course, I have not spent a lot of time actually verifying that last assertion, but the thought of a bear going "UGGGHHH" in the woods? Not a pretty picture!

"Normal" bowel movements are like art. Its value is usually most appreciated by its owner. In fact, in Europe, most bathrooms in Switzerland, Germany, and Austria have little shelves to catch the droppings so you can examine it before flushing. On the other hand, some of the public bathrooms in Italy have these two little places to place your feet and a hole in the floor. Italians want to just get rid of their poop as fast as they can.

What's so interesting about this dichotomy is that my Italian friends are only too happy to discuss bathroom activity and my German friends are incredibly reluctant. Talk about the yin and the yang.

It's important to pay attention to consistency, color, frequency, and the ease with which you go. The color of your poop is important, but you need to remember that it is also relative and very individual. (If your poop is black, it could indicate bleeding in your upper stomach. The poop turns black because the blood is dried by time you pass the stool. It can also signify an excessive amount of iron. Poop with red may indicate bleeding in the colon area, and clay in color indicates a possible liver impairment.) Keep in mind that you poop what you eat, so if you eat a lot of greens, it'll show in your poop. The smell of your bowel movement can also be an indicator of things gone awry. If it smells really bad, it can be an indicator of bacteria or some kind of infection. It can also be smelly because the excess waste has been sitting in your colon for a really long time. There are varying degrees of the odor. Sometimes you'll notice only a trace of that rotten-egg smell, and other times you can light all the matches you want, or spray air freshener like crazy, but you'll never kill that odor. The worse your poop smells, the more likely you're having digestive problems. Keep an eye out for any irregularities such as blood in your stool or unusual bouts of diarrhea or constipation. Contact your doctor immediately if you notice anything unusual. These irregularities can be very serious and should not be ignored.

Digestive Disorders

A number of symptoms can affect your normal regularity and the ease of your bowel movements. Most of these can be easily detected and treated if you know what to look for. Maintaining a proper and healthy diet will help significantly if you think you suffer from any of these disorders.

Digestive disorders afflict one out of every two Americans at some point. They result in thousands of absences from work on a daily basis and cost the nation $50 *billion* a year. That's *billion* with a "B"! It's not normal to have abdominal pain or to have your bowel movements interfere with your life. But statistics show that at some point you will be faced with the perils of some or maybe all of the following common digestive disorders. Usually (hopefully) you don't need to give a second thought to your digestion. It's as natural to us as breathing. But every now and then a rumble down below or a little excess wind from behind reminds us that we are human. Here's what you'll need to know, including symptoms, causes, and treatments.

Gas

Everyone gets gas. In fact, it has been said that it's the true test of a relationship. Can you easily and casually pass gas in front of your significant other? "Passing wind" or burping allows the body to get rid of extra gas, which is usually caused by excess swallowed air. Contrary to popular belief, foods like broccoli, beans, cabbage, and cauliflower, or even an increase in your fiber intake, do not cause gas. These foods have gotten a bad rap over the years, because it is actually the combination of those foods with other food you're eating that cause the reaction. (For more information on this refer to Chapter 9 on food combining). Any one of those foods alone will not cause gas, but miscombine food and you will have some problems. Flatulence is gas created through bacterial action in the bowel and is passed rectally. Ten to eighteen "breezes" a day are considered "normal," but they don't have to be that frequent. As you start eating a better diet, you'll find that the frequency is greatly lowered. Most people produce one to three pints of gas a day. Usually the gas is an odorless vapor made up of carbon dioxide, oxygen, nitrogen, hydrogen, and sometimes methane. On occasion, these vapors can really pack a punch because of bacteria in the large intestine that release small amounts of gases containing sulfur. It's also a good indication of bad food combining. At that moment, whether receiving or giving, you may not want to stand down wind. Trace gases related to certain foods you might have eaten often cause the noticeable smell. Excessive passing of gas could be due to a lactose intolerance. (This would be a superb reason to get off dairy products if this is of concern to you!) Certain starches could also trigger gas, like wheat, oats, corn, or even potatoes when combined with protein. And contrary to common advice, eating fruit after a meal will give you gas because it starts the fermentation process. If you suffer from bouts of gas, you may also notice some abdominal distention, bloating, and even discomfort. Pain and bloating can occur in the abdominal region when excess gas gathers in the digestive tract. Abdominal distention is usually worse at night and can be relieved by a yoga move I do. If you get on all fours, placing your elbows and fore-arms flat on the floor, you tush will naturally stick up in the air and your lower abdominal region will feel relief. It goes without saying that you'll probably want to do this exercise in private. (Unless of course, you don't mind sticking your butt in the air!) To avoid these symptoms, regular abdominal exercises such as sit-ups or stomach contractions several times a day will help. Avoiding irritating foods like those mentioned above will also help alleviate the distention and discomfort.

An occasional belch during or after a meal is normal, and in some countries a true testament of your appreciation for the chef's gastronomic fare. Eating or drinking too fast most commonly causes belching or burping, which is the other way your body can eliminate excess gas. Drinking carbonated beverages, chewing gum, sucking on hard candies, and excessive swallowing due to nervous tension are also common causes of burps. Avoid these culprits to eliminate excessive belching. If you notice an increase in the frequency of your belching, it might indicate an upper gastrointestinal disorder like a peptic ulcer, gastritis, or gastroesoph-ageal reflux disease (GERD). You should see your doctor immediately if you suspect any of these.

Although gas may be uncomfortable to you, it is surely not life-threatening. Besides, you can always blame it on the dog, right?

Constipation

An estimated 50 million Americans get "blocked up" on occasion. Eighteen million Americans, women twice as often as men, feel constipated on a regular basis. In 1993, Americans spent $740 million on over-the-counter laxatives. That doesn't include all the cups of coffee Americans drink on a daily basis to help get things moving right along! No wonder Starbucks is popping up on every corner!

Here's what you need to know. Constipation is defined as hard, dry, and often painful poop. If it looks like it belongs in kitty litter rather than your toilet, you're constipated. If the urge to go is less frequent than three times a week, you are constipated. Bowel movements can be affected by so many variables, including age, diet, and your regular cycle. Excess waste that is stored in the body gets absorbed and can be dangerous to your health. The most important thing to pay attention to is the ease with which you go and the shape of your stool. Constipation is a symptom and not a disease. It is caused by something else. Doctors aren't sure why women get constipated more than men, but they know that factors such as diet, dieting, pregnancy, menstrual cycle, and side effects from certain medicines are common causes. Antidepressants, medicines with codeine, and even iron and calcium supplements can cause constipation. Women are probably more uptight about going to the bathroom than men, too. Diets high in animal fat (meat, dairy, and eggs) and refined sugar (one of the most constipating foods, often found in rich desserts and candy), and diets low in fiber (vegetables, fruits, and whole grains), are believed to con-

tribute to constipation (maybe that's why women are more constipated than men). A sudden change in your regular routine can also
cause constipation, which is why you might find yourself "blocked"
while on vacation. You change your eating habits, drinking habits,
and even your sleep pattern. It makes sense, doesn't it? You can
even imagine constipation by *thinking* you have it, but the frequency with which you go is not as often as you thought. In fact, if
you ignore the urge to go long enough, you can and probably will
self-induce your constipation. Just reading this paragraph can cause
constipation! Some people ignore the urge to avoid using a public
bathroom (a real condition referred to as paruresis) or simply do
not make the time in their day to poop. After a while, you may no
longer feel the urge, and that can lead to progressive constipation.
Listen to me on this one. Don't miss your turn at bat. When you
gotta go . . . you gotta go! Chronic constipation can be a sign of
the onset of irritable bowel syndrome (IBS), which I will discuss
later in this chapter.

So what can you do to prevent this blockage? After all, unlike
some of us actors, the intestinal tract is not a demand performer.

The best advice I can offer you to combat constipation is to
improve the quality of your food, chew it well, properly combine
your food, add fiber to your diet, and drink enough water between
meals. Try to avoid a quick fix by using a laxative. Bears don't need
Ex-Lax. Nature takes its course if you have the right map. We're
natural healers, and I have found that if you just give people the
right information, they will respond to it brilliantly. Here's how
you can avoid and prevent constipation.

❋   ❋   ❋   ❋   ❋   ❋   ❋   ❋   ❋   ❋

TIPS TO AVOID CONSTIPATION:

- **Eat a well-balanced diet that includes whole grains, fresh fruits, bran, and vegetables.**
- **Drink plenty of fluids between meals, but avoid caffeine.**

- **Exercise regularly.**
- **Don't ignore your urge to go.**
- **Make time to go.**

❈   ❈   ❈   ❈   ❈   ❈   ❈   ❈   ❈   ❈

Diarrhea

The National Institutes of Health in Washington, D.C., estimate that Americans suffer through 99 million bouts of diarrhea a year. There are many causes, ranging from contaminated drinking water to improperly handled food. Travel, stress, lactose intolerance, antibiotics, antacids, caffeine, and artificial sweeteners can all trigger that grumble in your gut. Unlike constipation, women and men seem equally likely to have a run-in with the runs. Officially, diarrhea is defined as abnormal looseness of stools or an increase in the frequency of your bowel movements. Typically, diarrhea lasts no more than two to three days and doesn't merit a trip to the doctor. If the diarrhea lasts more than three weeks, it is classified as chronic, and you should definitely see your doctor.

So how do you get diarrhea, anyway? Usually it's caused by a viral or bacterial infection. The enormous amounts of watery poop you see are a result of toxins that are part of the bug invading your body. Women tend to have a higher rate of exposure to these transmitters of germs and viruses because they're around little kids more often. Believe it or not, kids are some of the best carriers of these critters. The best defense against diarrhea is to make sure you wash your hands . . . often.

Diarrhea can also be caused from mishandled or undercooked food. Bacterial infections in food account for between 6 million and 81 million cases of food poisoning a year in the United States, and 9,000 deaths, according to the Center for Disease Control.

Restoring lost fluids is key to your recovery from diarrhea. You want to stay properly hydrated so you don't get dizzy or, even worse, sicker. Water or juice is a good replacement, or even something like miso soup, which has amazing healing properties. You should avoid drinks with caffeine. Caffeine is a diuretic and will have the opposite effect from what you are seeking. It's also a good idea to eat foods that are easy for your system to digest, such as rice, dry toast, or a clear soup (like miso soup). One of the best foods for fighting diarrhea, especially for babies and children, is bananas. It's a good binding food and it replaces lost potassium. Carbohydrates help your intestine digest a little bit more easily. And as you well know by now, *NO DAIRY!*

Diarrhea is often brought on by travel. It's one of the most common health problems for frequent travelers. Too bad you can't get frequent flier miles for frequent trips to the toilet, huh? Each year 3 million to 5 million Americans visit developing countries, and 40–60 percent of these travelers will get diarrhea, or what is referred to as travelers' diarrhea. Taking proper caution while abroad will reduce your risk greatly. Bottled drinks, hot drinks, and foods you can easily identify are best choices. Tap water should always be avoided, even when brushing your teeth. Stay away from drinks with ice, too. It's also a good idea to stay away from raw veggies, lettuce that has a high water content, fruit, meat, shellfish, and food from street vendors.

Of all the problems associated with diarrhea, that sense of needing the bathroom right now may be the scariest. There's nothing worse than being out and getting that feeling in your gut and just knowing you're moments away from an "accident." This is called urgent diarrhea. And though it's really no different from any other diarrhea, it seems to come from nowhere, and always at the most inopportune times. Greasy, fatty foods are often the culprit, and alcohol can trigger this effect, too. You may even find that your body manifests stress by giving you a bout of the runs. I assure you that if you relieve that stress, your dash to the bathroom won't be nearly as often.

Irritable Bowel Syndrome/Inflammatory Bowel Disease

You'll know the second you experience any of the symptoms from these two gut-wrenching diseases. The pain will be so sharp in your belly that you'd make a deal with the devil himself to stop the burning and cramping. Oh, and after you feel the first onset of the pain, you'd better be near a bathroom, because you are only moments away from hatching what feels like an alien baby from your bottom. Irritable bowel syndrome (IBS) is a common intestinal disorder that leads to crampy pain, gassiness, bloating, and noticeable changes in your bowel habits. Some people experience diarrhea while others are constipated. Often, IBS will be a severe swing between the two. IBS has been called many things over the years: colitis, spastic colon, or functional bowel disease. These terms are not accurate for the symptoms. Colitis means an inflamed large intestine or colon; IBS does not cause inflammation and should not be confused. Doctors refer to IBS as a functional disorder, because there is no sign of disease when the colon is examined. Though IBS is quite uncomfortable, it does not cause any permanent harm to the intestines. It is believed that the main cause of IBS is stress. Researchers have found that a person who suffers from IBS has a colon that is more sensitive and reactive than usual. It begins to spasm after only mild stimulation, so ordinary activities such as eating, distention from gas, or other waste materials trapped in the colon can trigger a reaction. Chocolate, milk products, and excessive alcohol are frequent offenders. Caffeine, especially coffee, affects those with IBS more often, causing loose, watery stools. Someone who suffers from IBS can have the urge to go as quickly as thirty to sixty minutes after eating, which means you'd better not be too far from a bathroom, *ever!* The eating causes a contraction in the colon, and that triggers the urge, usually accompanied by really harsh cramps and diarrhea. The severity of the response usually depends on the number of calories and the amount of fat in the meal. Fat in any form is a strong stimulus of colon contractions after eating. Most foods we eat contain some fat, so just about anything can trigger a response.

Doctors don't completely understand why or how stress triggers the same type of colonic response, but it may be because the colon is partly controlled by the nervous system. Reducing the amount of stress can reduce the frequency of an IBS flare-up.

Eating a balanced diet can help lessen the symptoms of IBS. A good idea is to keep a food journal to document everything you eat and drink to determine whether anything in particular may be causing the reaction. You should discuss your findings with your doctor to determine if a simple change in your diet will solve the problem or whether you may need to be on medication to help control the situation. Dietary fiber may lessen the symptoms, too. High-fiber diets keep the colon slightly distended, which can help prevent spasms from occurring. Whole grain bread, cereals, beans, fruits, and vegetables are all good sources of fiber, or you can also take a fiber supplement. Sometimes excess fiber in your diet can cause gas, but that side effect ought to diminish within a few weeks. Try to maintain a balanced diet that is low in fat and high in carbohydrates for your best results.

IBS has not been proven to be linked to any serious organic diseases. There is no link between IBS and other inflammatory bowel diseases, such as Crohn's disease or ulcerative colitis. There is no medical proof that IBS leads to cancer. There are variations of severity of IBS, which may cause you to be sidelined for a while, but it is not a life-threatening disease.

Inflammatory bowel disease (IBD) is far more serious than IBS. IBD affects more than 1 million men and women in America, and 10–25 percent of the cases may have a genetic link. There can either be a glitch in the immune system or an inherited genetic defect. Jacqueline Wolf, M.D., assistant professor of Harvard Medical School and codirector of the IBD Center at Brigham and Women's Hospital in Boston, has a three-step theory on IBD. First, Dr. Wolf believes that a genetic disposition sets the stage. Then a virus or bacteria in the intestine penetrates the intestinal wall. Finally, the immune system goes on the attack and ends up destroying the intestine rather than the intruder. There are two types of IBD, which are identified by where the flare-up occurs and how deeply it affects the intestinal walls. Ulcerative colitis occurs when the inflammation moves up to the large intestine and sticks to the surface of your gut. It usually starts in the same place every time it flares, which is most commonly the lining of the rectum. The disease usually occurs between the ages of fifteen and thirty-five. Nausea, diarrhea, and severe pain are the common symptoms. Usually surgery to remove the infected area eliminates the disease. Crohn's disease occurs when the inflammation moves all around your stomach, and can involve the intestinal wall literally from your mouth to your tush. Crohn's is a particularly nasty disease. It causes nausea, vomiting, diarrhea (sometimes with blood in it), and tremendous abdominal pain. The disease can spread throughout the other areas in the region by passing through the intestinal wall and to other organs. It can lead to intestinal blockage, infertility, other infections, and even cancer. See your doctor right away if you suspect you may be experiencing any of these symptoms. This can be a very serious condition, especially if it goes untreated.

Unlike IBS, it will take more than reducing your stress level or changing your diet to handle the symptoms brought on by IBD. Of course, you still want to watch your diet, and your appetite may be diminished, so it's important that you focus on eating the right things. Dr. Wolf suggests a well-rounded diet consisting of fresh fruit, steamed fish and vegetables, and lots of carbohydrates. They will help prevent dehydration and malnutrition brought on by the severe weight loss. Dr. Wolf suggests keeping an eye out for foods that can trigger a reaction. Once again, a food journal will help you monitor those foods and effects. Unlike IBS, fiber should be used cautiously if you have IBD. Too much fiber can cause obstructions, particularly in bowel walls that might be swollen. Talk with your doctor about specific medications used to control the flare-ups associated with these two diseases. Also talk to your doctor if you are on birth control pills. There is some question whether birth control pills can trigger Crohn's in women who are already genetically predisposed to the disease.

IBD, ulcerative colitis, and Crohn's disease are not conditions to ignore. If you detect the symptoms, see your doctor at once. The diseases can be managed. You do not have to become incapacitated by IBD.

Heartburn

Late-night eating + a large meal + chock full of fat = ? What is this formula for, you ask? H-E-A-R-T-B-U-R-N! Do you remember those old Alka-Seltzer ads, "I can't believe I ate the whole thing"? Sure enough, you ate it, all right. Now what do you do? It tasted *soooo* good going down, but now you're paying the price.

What people eat and when they eat it are the most common causes of heartburn, also known as acid indigestion or a sour stomach. In fact, some people get such severe heartburn, they're certain they're suffering a heart attack. Heartburn occurs when gastric acid from the stomach backs up into the esophagus, causing irritation, inflammation, and even ulceration. If you eat too fast or miscombine food, you'll suffer. Some 75 million Americans get heartburn one or two times a month. Some 14 million Americans suffer from heartburn on a daily basis. The antacid business enjoys $2 billion to $3 billion in sales annually as a result. We should not accept heartburn as a way of life!

Fat, alcohol, smoking, and candy such as mints or chocolate can weaken the lower esophageal muscle that controls the opening between your stomach and your esophagus. This can cause an acid reflux, which in turn causes a burning sensation, chest tightness, and sometimes a feeling of warmth sweeping into the throat. Voilà! You've got heartburn. Eating large meals late at night increases the likelihood of the onset of such symptoms. Sometimes even aspirin or prescription drugs can bring on the fire.

You can take an antacid, but be aware that taking an antacid slows down the digestive process because antacids neutralize the digestive juices. It's really a vicious cycle that can be broken if you're eating right. For a natural alternative, you can try eating a papaya. Papayas contain the enzyme papain, which soothes the stomach. If you can't find fresh papaya, most health food stores sell papaya tablets, which are almost as good. Like all the digestive disorders I have discussed, eating a healthy diet can control heartburn. Certain foods, like onions and candy (especially chocolate and mints), as well as real fatty foods promote heartburn. Very acidic foods and juices can also cause these symptoms and can increase the severity of the pain, too. Tomatoes, citric fruit juices, spicy food, and even coffee are just a few of the foods you should avoid if you are prone to getting heartburn. Try not to eat late-night meals. If you eat right before going to bed, you're more likely to suffer. Lying down relaxes the esophagus, allowing acid to flow more easily. You should also avoid smoking and drinking alcoholic drinks, especially those mixed with fruit drinks like tomato, orange, or grapefruit juices. Excess weight can also trigger heartburn, so there's another reason to lose weight and feel great.

Fix It with Fiber

I've mentioned fiber a few times throughout this chapter, and it might be a good idea to expand on the benefits of a fiber-rich diet, or eating your "roughage," as Mom used to say. Fiber-rich foods, such as fresh fruits, vegetables, grains, and beans, increase the bulk and water content of your stools. The bigger and the wetter your poop, the more easily and quickly it should pass through your intestines.

Most Americans don't eat enough fiber, and it's one of the best weapons in the arsenal to fight aging. Fiber is the front runner in fighting heart disease, breast and other cancers, high cholesterol, high blood pressure, and many of the digestive disorders we discussed earlier in this chapter. Fiber will help keep your body running like the well-oiled machine it was meant to be. The National Cancer Institute recommends getting twenty to thirty grams of fiber a day. Most Americans eat only one-third that amount. You can take fiber supplements such as Metamucil to boost your daily fiber intake if you're not already eating enough fiber-rich foods. But remember, there's no nutrient content in a supplement, so it's better to try to maintain a fiber-filled food selection.

So what is fiber made of, anyway? It's a complex mixture of indigestible substances that makes up the structural material of plants. There are very few calories in fiber, and it isn't a source of energy for your body. It does not get broken down like other foods we ingest. What fiber does do for you, though, is carry away bad guys like cholesterol and other toxins out of your system. It's like having little scrub bubbles to clean up the wall of your colon. The term *roughage* comes from insoluble fiber, which truly cleans out your system. It absorbs water and helps make your poop softer and easier to pass. Eating this type of fiber helps conditions like constipation and IBS. Soluble fibers, on the other hand, dissolve in water, and become sticky inside your body. As they pass through your system, they pick up bile acids and other toxins and cart those bad guys out of there. Bran, which is the coarse outer layer of wheat, rice, oats, and corn, has the highest concentration of fiber. That's why all the healthy breakfast cereals these days are bran-based in nature. In fact, Michael H. Davidson, M.D., medical director of the Chicago Center for Clinical Research at Rush Presbyterian–St. Luke's Hospital, says that eating just two ounces of oat bran a day is enough to lower your LDL cholesterol level 10–15 percent. Wheat bran is ideal for people with digestive disorders because it is a terrific source of insoluble fiber. It's the most common bran found in breakfast cereals. If you don't eat cereal, you can always try a bran muffin or bran bread as another good source of fiber.

Fiber does your body loads of good. It lowers cholesterol, because soluble fiber carries bile out of our digestive tract. It draws the so-called bad cholesterol (LDL cholesterol) out of the bloodstream and converts it to more bile, which it flushes away. Fiber reduces your risk of heart disease by lowering your cholesterol. The likelihood of heart attacks and strokes is also diminished by eating a high-fiber diet because it helps lower blood pressure, too. Many doctors believe eating insoluble fiber may be the key in the fight against breast cancer because it reduces estrogen levels (high levels of estrogen in women are believed to lead to breast cancer). In fact, fiber reduces your risk for colon and rectal cancer, too.

> *Too little fiber produces constipation and straining on the toilet, which may be a main cause of varicose veins.*

Fiber increases the level of acidity in the colon, making it an unfriendly home to cancer-causing toxins. Therefore, it helps stools pass more quickly through the system and won't allow it to spend a lot of unnecessary time in your colon to mix with any nasty carcinogens. It's like having the best garbage bags (double-thick handy bags) to carry all the waste and garbage out of your body.

Diabetes can be helped by eating fiber because it controls blood sugar and reduces the need for insulin. It delays the emptying of the stomach, which causes the sugars in food you eat to be absorbed more slowly. Finally, weight loss is helped by a fiber-rich diet because you'll naturally eat less fat in your diet. Fiber foods require you to eat more slowly and reduce your caloric intake because they naturally have fewer calories. Bottom line: Fiber is a good thing.

FIBER

Food	Portion	Fiber (grams)
Barley, pearled	½ cup	12.3
Pears, dried	5 halves	11.5
Health Valley Fruit & Fitness Cereal	¾ cup	11.0
Blackberries	1 cup	7.2
Chickpeas	½ cup	7.0
Kidney beans	½ cup	6.9
Lima beans	½ cup	6.8
Refried beans, canned	½ cup	6.7

Black beans	½ cup	6.1
Raspberries	1 cup	6.0
Whole-wheat spaghetti	1 cup	5.4
Figs, dried	3	5.2
Lentils	½ cup	5.2
Succotash	½ cup	5.2
Guava	1	4.9
Navy beans	½ cup	4.9
Artichoke hearts	½ cup	4.4
Pear	1	4.3
Oatmeal	½ cup	3.9
Raisins	½ cup	3.9
Wheat germ, toasted	¼ cup	3.7
Brussels sprouts	½ cup	3.4
Sweet potato	1	3.4
Orange	1	3.1
Apple	1	3.0

By now you've either put this book back on the bookshelf and think I'm a total nut, or, I hope, you now know how to respond when someone asks you, "What's the poop?" I really believe that all of this information is imperative to gauging your overall state of health. Once you know what you're supposed to be doing, you can acknowledge that you could be functioning more efficiently. Maintaining good eating habits can relieve every digestive disorder I mentioned. We put premium gas into our cars. We change the oil every 3,000 miles. What have you done for yourself lately?

18 | Listening to Your Body

Self-awareness is the beginning of wisdom and a prerequisite for self-care. In the crazy hustle and bustle of everyday life, we sometimes forget to be good listeners. The key to understanding other people is being able to listen to what they're telling you. Listening to yourself may be even more important. If you don't listen to your body for your health's sake, you could miss an important point, one that might someday save your life. When I was in Italy in 1982, I experienced a unique opportunity to sharpen my senses other than my speaking skills, because I didn't speak Italian (except *"senza formaggio"* which means "without cheese"!). Yet, through my observations of what was going on around me, I became more aware of nonverbal signals. Granted, these signals are always being sent to us, but because we normally have the ability to communicate through words, we don't pay as close attention to them. All of this nonverbal communication sparked the thought that if other people are sending messages without speaking, then I must be doing the same thing. I started to look beyond the surface in all communication. I looked for the more subtle messages both outside myself and then within. I made up my mind that I really wanted to *listen to my body*. There were probably messages all along that I wasn't even aware of! From then on, I decided that I would listen to these signals. I would sleep when I was tired, I would eat only when I was hungry, and I would stop eating when I was full. I paid attention to the foods I really wanted to eat and the effect of those conscious choices. I even began to notice the subtle fluctuations throughout my menstrual cycle. (I got so good at this that years later I knew exactly the moment I got pregnant with my two sons!) It was so amazing for me, because this was really the first time I consciously tried to pay attention and listen to what my body was telling me. I would analyze the cause and the effect of everything having to do with my health and well-being. I came home from Italy seven weeks later, thinner, healthier, well-rested, and with a bad Italian perm (I guess I hadn't learned to listen to my hair!).

Listening to your body is a sure way to start a program of preventive medicine, and it's something I encourage each and every person who reads my book to do. You don't want to have to start listening when it might be too late to fix the problem. So many people don't start thinking about their health until something happens that jolts them out of their lazy, unhealthy habits: a physician's grim diagnosis during a routine checkup or some chronic problem that becomes so unbearable, you have to finally face it. You're never too young or too old to start thinking about your health and listening to your body. I can't tell you how many friends laughed at me years ago for all my health follies, which seemed so eccentric at the time. So much of what I was talking about then has been proven medically and has become mainstream today. My friends aren't laughing anymore.

Listening to your body isn't just about "bad" things that might be going on. Have you ever had a "craving" for something a little "devilish" in the afternoon? Who hasn't had a sudden attack of *needing* a chocolate bar or salty potato chips every now and then? Food cravings can convey an important message from your body that something is out of balance. You may want to look at the food you've eaten before your craving to give you the answer, but it may be tied to emotional things instead. There's been so much written about the connection between food and mood (choosing chocolate because the serotonin replicates the feeling of falling in love, choosing nuts when you're angry because it allows you to vent your aggression with every crunch, comfort food chosen during times of stress because it's how your mother soothed you, and the list goes on and on). Antsy behavior or nervous shaking is another sign that you are out of balance, but it doesn't necessarily indicate a threat to your health. It could be too much caffeine. You may suffer symptoms of PMS before your period. Your body alerts you to the onset of your period by manifesting those symptoms. But you know that these cravings, mood swings, and bloating will go away. Likewise, you can get the same kind of information for many common ailments, if you're listening to what your body is saying. If something doesn't "feel right," your body will send you a message. It's up to you to pay attention to those messages and know how to interpret them. Pain, swelling, aching, nausea, breakouts, a stuffy nose, or even a chronic cough are all symptoms of something else that is wrong in your system or something you are allergic to in your environment. Tuning in to your body and its needs not only makes you feel better, but it can help you break unproductive habits that are more than likely undermining your health. As my father always said, "Anything that suggests a problem, is a problem."

By now, I've probably jarred some thoughts in your head about your health and your lifestyle. Maybe you haven't completely made up your mind that it's time to make some changes, and that's okay. But you can at least start paying attention to what your body is telling you. If a symptom is chronic or recurring you should definitely see your physician. If you are paying close enough attention, you ought to be able to determine the difference between a mild symptom and a major concern. Listening to your body will put you in charge of your health because you can work *with* your doctor instead of walking into his office saying, "Something's wrong, fix me!" Think of you and your doctor as a team.

The doctor is an expert in medicine, and you're an expert on your body. And after all, it's *your* body.

How to Set Up and Keep a Lifestyle Journal

We've all heard about the benefits of keeping a journal. You can keep a journal on absolutely everything. Throughout this book I have talked about keeping various personal journals to help you identify and manage body ailments and conditions. If you haven't tried detailing your activities on a daily basis by recording them in a notebook, diary, or journal, you don't know what you're missing. I mean you *really don't know* what you're missing, because there could be telltale signs of something going on in your body or with your health that you just can't see unless you are tracking several aspects of your life. Keeping a lifestyle journal allows you to track the six essential areas of your life. Not only will you be able to chart the constants in your day-to-day life, you will be able to spot and (I hope) prevent health issues before they become bigger problems.

This all seems a little obsessive at first, but in actuality, it shouldn't take more than a few minutes of your time each day. I recommend that you do it for the first three months when starting the program. Here's an example of what I put in my lifestyle journal.

DAY OF CYCLE	DATE	EXERCISE	FOOD/ DRINK	SLEEP	BATHROOM	WEIGHT
14	1/31/98	2 miles	see food journal	6 hours	2M	122
15	2/1/98	2.5 miles	see food journal	5.5 hours	2M	121

Tracking Your Weight

Keep track of your (true) weight, but you don't have to be fanatical about it. So many elements can affect your weight, and as most of you know, it can vary by five pounds (or more) on a daily basis. Water retention, a sodium-heavy meal the night before, the onset of your period, flying, and even stress can all affect your weight. But if you're the kind of person who likes to know how much they weigh (I am) you can track your weight by two methods. You can keep a weight journal, weighing yourself often and recording your weight, allowing you to understand the daily fluctuations. Or you can go by the way your clothes fit. You can tell if your favorite pair of jeans feel tight or loose, and use that as a barometer. I've used both exclusively, and now use both concurrently. If you're choosing the "scale" method, it's good to weigh yourself often and write it down to be able to see on paper the ebb and flow of your body and its cycle. After three months of keeping a weight journal, you'll be so aware of how your body feels at a certain weight that you'll be able to guess your weight before you even get on the scale. I always know what I'm going to see on that scale because I know how my body feels to me. Some experts tell you to weigh yourself on the same day and at the same time every week. That never worked for me because the day before the weigh-in could be different from week to week, and the number on the scale wouldn't be indicative of my true weight.

If you don't want to weigh yourself for fear of being tied to a number on the scale (AKA fatsophobia numerosis), then use how your clothing fits as your guide (Deepak Clothesa). The only danger in this method is with all the loose clothing and Lycra we wear, by the time you feel you've put on a few pounds, it's more like ten.

What to Put in Your Journal

❋ Your weight.

Tracking Your Food

Keeping track of everything you eat on a daily basis is one of the best tools you can use to get control over your eating. So often, people will pop a few peanuts, pretzels, M&Ms, or what have you, into their mouth and it's practically an unconscious action. People trick themselves into believing they're not really eating if they're standing up. Or they become victims of what I call the Mommy Syndrome, which is "I'm not *really* eating. I'm just finishing what the kids left on their plates." We all do it, and most of the time we're not even aware of it. Maybe you're a mid-afternoon or late-night snacker, and because it wasn't exactly a meal (it was the left-over pizza slice or the rest of your pasta from last night), you hardly count it as a meal. Writing down every single thing you put into your mouth will help you realize the amount of food you actually consume.

It can also help if you suspect that a certain symptom might be related to something you're eating. You should include all new foods that you introduce to your system. Say you've never tried sushi before. Make a note that it was the first time you ate raw fish. See if there is any correlating symptom that arises from trying this new food. Remember that you are the boss over what you eat each and every day. You can't focus on what might be wrong with your diet unless you really know your habits. We are creatures of habit, and sometimes, we aren't even aware of things we do, like eating. Writing down everything you eat will help you focus in on those areas that could stand a little improvement and let you know the areas you're doing just fine in too!

> *Take a real look at how you're eating. Keep a journal. Write everything down. It's a really concrete way to understand why you feel terrible the day after eating something heavy or poorly food combined.*
>
> LILLIE KAE STEVENS, ACTRESS

237

Food Allergies and Food Intolerances

What most people call a food allergy is really a food intolerance, which is an entirely different ailment. In fact, food allergies are far less common than people think.

An allergy to food develops when a person's immune system mistakes a food, drink, condiment, spice, flavoring, or preservative for a dangerous foreign invader. The body manufactures special antibodies to repel any subsequent "invasion." The next time you eat that particular food, those antibodies are going to trigger a chemical attack as their response. The fallout tends to come quickly, usually within minutes and almost always within a few hours. Symptoms can include swelling of the lips; numbness or tingling of the mouth; itching; a rash; a runny nose; intestinal pain, cramping, gas, diarrhea, nausea, or even vomiting; and sometimes wheezing and a shortness of breath. The most severe cases can cause respiratory arrest.

> *Food allergies affect 1 to 2 percent of the U.S. population (2.5 million to 5.2 million Americans).*

The foods that most often cause allergies in adults are dairy, nuts, shellfish, yeast, and gluten (found in oats, barley, rye, and wheat). Dairy is a biggie in my family. You can build up to what looks like an allergic reaction to food (but is really an intolerance to it), so you should try to vary the foods you eat on a regular basis.

There's no real treatment for food allergies, except to stop eating those offending foods. This means carefully reading labels, interrogating your waiters, and avoiding potentially spoiled and dangerous foods. (Well, that last one is a good idea for everyone!)

An intolerance to food means your body isn't biologically equipped to handle a certain food or additive. It has nothing to do with the immune system. Symptoms usually appear within twelve hours after the offending food is consumed. The most common symptoms are digestive complaints, including bloating, diarrhea, gas, heartburn, or nausea. High-fiber foods, such as beans, bran, and vegetables like broccoli, cabbage, brussels sprouts, and cauliflower, are thought to be hard to tolerate for some people. I, of course contend that it is not those foods individually, but the

About 30 million Americans are lactose intolerant.

foods you eat in combination with those foods that causes the discomfort and intolerance. Another good example is someone who is lactose intolerant, which is when the body lacks the enzyme that breaks down the sugar in milk. Some people have a hard time tolerating foods that have a druglike agent such as caffeine. Chocolate and cheese products have amines in them and are known to cause headaches. Certain foods can provoke a response in people with peptic ulcers or intestinal and digestive disorders.

Even the most health-conscious person can unknowingly (or at least unintentionally) eat something that's bound to have an adverse effect sooner or later. Though many might overlook their response, a serious reaction to a food allergy or intolerance can be debilitating and, for a few, even deadly. People with true food allergies must avoid the offending foods at all times. People with food intolerances may be able to eat an offending food, but only in a small portion and on a rare occasion. (You may want to ask yourself, before indulging in a food you know you can't tolerate, "Is it worth the headache? Is it worth the runny nose?") The greatest concern for people with a food allergy is anaphylaxis, which is a life-threatening reaction to an offending food. An anaphylactic reaction starts with itchy skin around the mouth and eyes, and can cause swollen lips and mouth. It progresses to breathing difficulties, a severe drop in blood pressure, unconsciousness, and in worst cases, death. This horrific chain of events can start within minutes of eating a food you are allergic to, and can last for several hours afterward. Immediate medical attention is required for those who suffer an anaphylactic reaction. Fortunately, this type of reaction is rare and can be avoided by eliminating foods you are allergic to. People with extreme food allergies have to be very savvy about their food choices. Injectable epinephrine, a synthetic version of a naturally occurring hormone called adrenaline, is used to treat anaphylactic shock. It is injected straight into a muscle or vein and goes right to the cardiovascular and respiratory systems, causing rapid constriction of blood vessels, relaxing lung muscles, reversing throat swelling, making it easier for the victim to breathe. It comes by prescription in two forms for home use, EpiPen (a premeasured single dose of epinephrine that comes in an automatic injector) or Ana-Kit (a traditional needle and syringe kit that comes with two doses). Those with serious food allergies should carry one of these with them at all times in case an anaphylactic reaction occurs.

The new labeling changes make it easier for food allergy sufferers to readily identify those foods that could contain ingredients that will cause a reaction. Originally, food standards were adopted to ensure uniformity. Today, ingredients are listed on labels because that is what is in that product. If you have a food allergy, you really have to alter your life. Remember that the majority of people who suffer from a food allergy are allergic to three or fewer foods. Adapting your lifestyle to avoid these foods is easy compared to suffering the consequences of eating them. Read your labels carefully so that you don't have a severe reaction. Knowing what foods to avoid will become part of your regular daily activity. The bummer is not knowing you have an allergy (or have had an allergy for years) and continuing unknowingly to suffer. Keeping track of the food you eat, as discussed in this chapter, will definitely help you identify any foods that may be causing you problems.

What to Put in Your Journal

❋ Write down everything you eat and drink every day. Include portion size. (Remember the old rule that 3.3 ounces of meat, chicken, or fish are approximately equal to the size of a deck of cards.) If you don't know exact portion size, make an estimate.

❋ Write down the time of day you eat.

❋ Don't forget to write down snacks, tastes, and a handful of peanuts. *Everything counts!*

❋ Note any effects of your eating, such as gas, diarrhea, constipation, and other gastrointestinal reactions. Also note any intolerances or allergic reactions.

Tracking Your Exercise

Record all exercise activity. It's a real key to staying fit and healthy. Of course, 20 minutes of aerobic activity three times a week is the minimum amount of exercise you need to keep fit. I'm recommending that you do something (even for a short time) to break a sweat *every day*. Remember to include exercise you get in addition to going to the gym, like a walk after dinner, skiing, or racquetball. They all count!

What to Put in Your Journal

❋ All exercise activity.
❋ Duration of activity.

Tracking Your Bathroom Activity

In Chapter 17, I explain the reasons behind keeping track of your bathroom activity. It's important to track your regularity (or irregularity) to make sure your body is properly functioning as it should.

What to Put in Your Journal

* Write down the time of the activity.

* Make a note if you feel any pain or discomfort.

* Take a look after you go. Notice if there are any irregularities floating (or sunk) that should be of concern. Any abnormal discoloration or odors should be noted.

Tracking Your Sleep

Sleep is a particular area in which your body shouts back and says, "I need rest!" If you deprive yourself of the much-needed time to rejuvenate your body, you'll be paying the price sooner or later (probably sooner), and one way or another (probably your health). Some people can systematically fall asleep, while others have a much harder time catching some zzz's. Keeping track of your sleep patterns will help you identify the cause of your insomnia or the reason you tossed and turned after eating that late-night snack.

What to Put in Your Journal

* Calculate the number of hours each night you actually sleep. (Tossing and turning don't count.)

* Keep track of the number of times you wake up during the night.

❋ Write down whether you were sleepy the next day, and whether you took a nap.

Tracking Your Menstrual Cycle

If you're a woman, every month from puberty until the aftermath of menopause, your body goes through a natural cleansing process known as your menstrual cycle. The monthly cycle can be different for everyone, so keeping a journal will help you understand what is regular for *you*. Weight gain or loss can affect your cycle, as can stress and travel. A change in your normal day-to-day activities can cause a reaction resulting in a variation from your regular schedule. Any deviation in your cycle could indicate that something is out of balance. Keeping track of all of these elements will help you identify the probable cause of such unbalances.

What to Put in Your Journal

❋ Write down the day of your current cycle.

❋ Note any symptoms such as PMS, cramping, and breakouts. Note any irregularities, such as missing your period or excessive and unusual bleeding.

Professional athletes stay very attuned to listening to their bodies. They have to keep themselves in world-class condition. Their main goal is to eat the right foods to be energetic at the right times, and to know which foods to avoid that might put a damper on their performance. Physically, they train to stay strong and keep up their endurance. They practice their sport day in and day out. Emotionally, they are aware of issues that might be acting as a mental block or psychological weight that might be holding them back from performing at their peak. They listen to their body when it talks. Joint pain, cramping, soreness, constipation, and diarrhea are all indicators that the athlete is pushing the body to the limit. Awaken the athlete that lives within each and every one of you. You don't have to run marathons or ski in the downhill championship. The Masters Golf Tournament and Wimbledon probably aren't in most of our futures. But without your health, you are not even in your *own* future. Don't ignore what your body is telling you. Be there for your body, and your body will surely be there for you. It's *your* future, *your* body, *your* health, and *your* happiness. BE THERE!

19 | Alternative/ Preventive Medicine

First do no harm.
HIPPOCRATES

There's been an enormous amount of Eastern influence throughout this book. Traditional Eastern medicine emphasizes integrity of human mind and body, and the interaction with the natural and social environments. It recognizes the importance of physical, nutritional, psychological, and spiritual factors in health. Its focus is on health promotion and preventive care. Some well-known traditional Chinese medicines that are practiced in Western countries are acupressure, acupuncture, herbal supplements, as well as relaxation exercises and techniques like tai chi, yoga, and meditation. At the center of these practices is the concept of qi (chi) or "vital energy." Qi is the ability to maintain harmony and keep the yin and yang in perfect balance. (This is also known as "Prana" in India, French philosopher Henri Bergson called it "Elan Vital," and well-known Western psychoanalyst Wilhelm Reich called it "Orgone Energy.") Regardless of what you want to call it, it is the *life force.* Recall from Chapter 2 that balance equals health. Imbalance results in sickness. Eastern medicine moves an out-of-balance body into balance and a state of qi. Many Western doctors see traditional Asian medicine as nonscientific, low technology, and based on ideas with no proven efficacy. But most people who try any of these methods believe in them because they work and bring results.

New York Times reporter James Reston is generally credited with introducing traditional Chinese Medicine (particularly acupuncture) to the West. While covering President Nixon's trip to China in 1971, Mr. Reston had to undergo emergency surgery to remove his appendix. He was treated with acupuncture for postsurgical pain. He went on to write a front-page story for the *Times* on his experience, proclaiming, "I've seen the past, and it works!"—a headline so bold, it grabbed the attention of many Western doctors who were eager to study the claims

A study reported in the 1993 New England Journal of Medicine showed that one out of every three Americans had tried an alternative medicine treatment in the previous year.

Reston made and the virtues of acupuncture. The research showed that traditional Chinese medicine takes a holistic approach based on the idea that no single part of the body can be understood, except in its relationship to the whole. The Eastern doctor looks at symptoms, lifestyle, diet, environmental influences, and other aspects of life that may be out of balance.

Authors such as Deepak Chopra have brought the ideas of India-based medicinal practices, known as "Ayurvedic" medicine, into vogue in recent years with best-selling books. The basis of this practice suggests that health is cultivated from an inner intelligence and a dynamic life force. Deepak Chopra's theories aim at restoring health by restoring balance, enhancing vitality, and living in harmony with surroundings. He believes that people have tremendous power over their health and well-being. And you do. It's a complete mind and body connection.

East Versus West

Though there is serious doubt that the two very different worlds of Eastern medicine and Western medicine will ever merge, the ideal scenario is to take the best of both worlds and develop a comprehensive, safe, and socially responsible approach to health care. The two worlds are so different (in areas such as diagnosis, treatment, even classification of diseases) that total integration would be impossible. The heart of practicing Eastern medicine is in taking care of one's self, both inner and outer. Self-awareness, relaxation, stress reduction, diet, and exercise are all elements that figure prominently into the healing process. A doctor practicing Western medicine will spend around fifteen minutes on a consultation with a patient. An Eastern doctor will spend almost an hour. (The diagnosis of a patient is more elaborate and extensive, and a thorough examination is necessary to find the "core" of the ailment. It involves looking, listening, smelling, asking questions, checking the tongue and the pulse.) Harriet Beinfeld, coauthor of *Between Heaven and Earth*, puts it this way: "Western doctors are like hunters, they identify and isolate a sickness, and take it out. Eastern doctors are more like gardeners; they nurture the body and help it thrive." Many patients derive a deep satisfaction from Eastern practices, as they become more in touch with their body through these healing methods.

In 1990, the cost of patient care for people with chronic illness and conditions was $659 billion. In 1993, the amount of money patients spent on alternative medicine was $14 billion.

Don't get me wrong on my thoughts regarding Western medicine. It is responsible for saving millions of lives, especially when it comes to emergency health care. But my focus is on prevention. It is B.E.S.T. when the two schools of thought can work together. For chronic, ongoing illness that creates everyday pain and suffering, I find that Eastern medicine offers a holistic and more reliable answer without the use of synthetic drugs or other artificial elements I don't want (or need) floating around in my bloodstream.

Alternative Medicines and Treatments: Do They Work?

The following is a list of alternative treatments that have been around for centuries and have now become mainstream medicinal practices. Perhaps you have heard of some of these but might not be familiar with exactly what they are. Here is a short description of each.

Acupuncture

A medical therapy developed in China more than 2,000 years ago, acupuncture is a method of pricking the skin or tissues with needles to treat various conditions. The premise is that all diseases cause a corresponding part of the body, called an acupuncture point, to become inflamed. The inflammation disappears when the condition is cured. The acupuncture point is found by dividing the body into "life and energy" channels called meridians. There are six main meridians, which correlate to approximately 1,000 acupuncture points. The channels are divided between the central nervous system and the circulatory system, and they might overlap in certain areas in common organs, but they are quite separate in the practice of acupuncture. The needles that are used are very very

> *Modern versions of acupuncture use electricity, heat, laser beams, sonar rays, and other nonneedle acupoint stimulators.*

fine, and though a lot of people get nervous about being pricked by a needle, if acupuncture is performed properly, you shouldn't feel any pain from the puncture. The needles are inserted and rotated gently and remain in position a few seconds to several minutes. Acupuncture is very mainstream in China and other Eastern countries. Acupuncture has become so much a part of accepted medical practices in the United States that there are twenty-one accredited schools and colleges in this country offering classes in acupuncture, and twelve more that offer accredited certification for practitioners (a license is a requirement for practitioners in this country). Acupuncture is often used in connection with herbal medicine.

Shiatsu and Acupressure

Shiatsu is the use of touch to stimulate and alter the flow of qi in the body to effectively cure whatever ails it. Shiatsu places pressure on any of the body's pressure points (usually by the thumbs) along the meridians to stimulate the flow of the life force, causing a cure for the illness, aches, and pains. It's known for its tremendous success in treating chronic headaches (especially migraines), back pain, and digestive problems. Acupressure is almost identical to shiatsu, except that the duration of the pressure is longer. Using acupressure can effectively treat ailments such as exhaustion, stomach disease, high blood pressure, nausea, sinus and nasal congestion, facial tension, and even toothaches.

Homeopathic Medicine

This philosophy is based on a simple premise: Less is more. Developed about 200 years ago by a German doctor named Samuel Hahnemann, homeopathic medicine has been widely practiced in Europe, Asia, and South America. Its foundation is the theory that "like cures like," and therefore the *cause* is often the *cure* to an ailment. A good example is the homeopathic use of a red onion to help relieve symptoms brought on by allergies. Cutting an onion causes watery eyes, a runny nose, and sneezing, which mimic the symptoms of an allergy. Instead of suppressing symptoms, homeopathic remedies mimic the symptoms and stimulate the body's defenses.

Homeopathic remedies are made by dissolving herbs, minerals, and certain animal extracts in an extremely diluted solution. "Potentization" consists of serial dilution of the active ingredient and shaking the combination. Potentization is believed to release a drug's curative energy while reducing its ability to cause an adverse reaction. The process of shaking and diluting the active ingredient can be repeated hundreds of times before the remedy is ever used, diluting it to such a point that the final product often has no measurable amount of the original medicinal substance.

The dilemma of homeopathic practices is that no one is exactly sure why these diluted remedies work. The concoctions mimic the symptoms of a disease but not the cause. Most believe that homeopathy works because it mixes the beliefs of traditional Chinese medicine and Ayurvedic traditions. Because a lot of the remedies are mostly water, some scientists and doctors think that the remedies work because the patients *will* themselves back to health through the power of the mind.

When making a diagnosis, a homeopath will take into consideration outside factors that may be adding to the symptoms, such as stress or the weather. Ailments such as allergies, arthritis, headaches, the flu, and respiratory infections are all successfully treated by this method. Homeopathic remedies can easily be found in most pharmacies and health food stores. You should see a homeopathic doctor for a proper diagnosis and remedy. Every homeopathic doctor I've ever seen has also been a medical doctor, but that is not always the case. Check out the credentials of whom you are seeing.

Alternative medicine is a healthy and pure approach to healing and health. Although the medical community in this country carefully scrutinizes these practices, there is no arguing with results. Patients who are interested in alternative medicine should give it a try. You'll want to make sure that you see an accredited practitioner and that you check his or her references, as you would for any doctor.

Herbs/Supplements

Let food be your medicine and medicine be your food.

HIPPOCRATES

I had never really committed to the whole vitamin and supplement thing prior to my pregnancy because I felt I was eating all the right foods and didn't need any supplementation to my diet or for my overall health. Doctors and nutritionists had often recommended a vitamin program, telling me to "take four of these and six of those." I used to buy those little plastic packs that had these huge "horse pill" size vitamins. But eventually my body just couldn't break the vitamins down, and they would pass whole. I would see these pills in my stool. They made me feel bloated and left a really metallic taste in my mouth. Then when I was pregnant with Nicky, I had to take prenatal vitamins. The original prescription from my doctor was terrible, but I had to take some vitamins, so I went to the health food store and found cap-

> *More than thirteen vitamins and twenty-two minerals are essential for normal body function.*

sulated prenatal vitamins that were great. I took some extra folic acid and calcium, too, and they worked like a charm. After I gave birth, I liked the idea of staying on the vitamins, so I started researching companies until I found a product that I could easily digest that fulfilled my supplemental needs. (In fact, I love the product so much, I am now a national spokesperson for the company!)

By taking vitamins and supplements, you are merely helping your body along and strengthening it if you have a deficiency. Your body needs a vitamin supplement if you are not getting enough nutritional absorption from the foods you eat. Either the food lacks the right vitamins, or your body is not absorbing the contents properly, or you don't chew your food enough to release the vitamins from the food. The massive amount of refinement and processing that most foods go through before we eat them greatly reduces the original vitamin content as well. Having a vitamin deficiency has been linked to such behavior as overeating, eating too fast, late-night eating, using caffeine, smoking, and eating a rich diet consisting of greasy, spicy, and/or high fat foods. Eating highly refined foods, such as foods that contain refined sugar or white flour, can effectively destroy essential nutrients in your body. Chemical additives and preservatives have also been shown to prohibit absorption.

It's virtually impossible to ensure that everything we eat is as vitamin-rich as it can be. We eat in restaurants, we eat in other people's homes, and unless we live on an organic farm, we can't get all our vitamins from food. Eliminating the negative foods from your diet and replacing them with vitamin-rich healthy and nutritious foods will greatly cut your need to use supplements. People who do choose to supplement their diet as a means to prevent disease and maintain their health cite the lack of proper nutrition in the food that's available, stress in their lives, and toxins used in the preservation of their food as the main reasons they take vitamins. It's a form of preventive medicine, but taking vitamins is not a cure for disease. The safest route for prevention is to avoid nutritional pitfalls and extremes. Eating a balanced (centered) diet that is properly food combined and is lacking in the unhealthy toxic waste some call food is your best weapon against disease and illness. Vitamins also provide the only source of certain coenzymes necessary for metabolism, the biochemical process that supports life.

Although we all hear the term "antioxidants" used so often these days, you might not know exactly what they are and do. They are supposed to be a great weapon in the war to reduce heart disease and cancer. Antioxidants are vitamins that enhance your body's ability to ward off free-radicals, which are unstable, hyperactive atoms in your body that do damage to your healthy cells and tissues. Eating foods that are rich in these antioxidant vitamins (C, E, and beta-carotene) is thought to be one way to protect yourself from heart disease, cancer, cataracts, immune deficiencies, and exercise-induced free-radical damage (caused by increased free-radical levels in the body after vigorous exercise).

Marilu's Secret Cure-alls

I have gathered some unusual and extremely useful cure-alls over the past nineteen years. All these are natural remedies for everyday common ailments. I've included them in this chapter because they are a form of alternative medicine, and they are remedies I really use. I have shared these secrets with friends for years, and now I get to share them with you. Hey, don't knock 'em till you try 'em!

Cold Sores

Cold sores usually indicate an imbalance of argenine to lysine in your system (two amino acids that work hand in hand). Too much argenine can be created in the body from eating foods that contain an abundance of argenine, such as peppers, potatoes, eggplant, tomatoes, and peanuts. The sun and stress can also create an over-production of argenine in the system. The best thing to do if you are prone to cold sores is to take 500 milligrams of lysine on a daily basis. At the first sign of a breakout, it is best to take 2,000 milligrams of lysine and to open a capsule and put the contents directly on the tender site.

Colds

If you think you've been exposed to a cold, or find yourself run down or caught in a drafty situation, the best thing to do is put your feet in the hottest water you can tolerate, soaking them for fifteen minutes. Remove them and quickly put on two pairs of thick socks and warm pajamas, cover your head, and get into bed. Take echinacea and goldenseal as directed on the bottle.

Headaches

I have few different remedies depending on what kind of headache you have. If your headache is in the front part of your head (yin headache from too much sugar, alcohol, etc.), the best remedy is a yang food like miso soup, or, in a pinch, tomato juice would balance it out. If your headache is in the back of your head (yang headache caused from stress, too much protein, etc.), a yin food like fruit juice or ginger will help get rid of that pounding in your head.

Jet Lag

I figured this one out when I went to Australia in 1987. Five days before you go someplace that is in a different time zone, figure out the time when you would be awake in both time zones, and eat protein and/or drink caffeine only in that common awake time. The rest of the time, eat only simple and carbohydrate meals. For example, if you live in New York and you're going to Rome (six hours later), stop eating protein and caffeine before 4 P.M. New York time. This includes eating on the plane. As soon as you arrive, do some light form of exercise and get on your new schedule.

Morning Sickness

I read that morning sickness occurs because of a 2 A.M. drop in calcium that our systems usually experience. Whenever I started to feel the slightest tinge of nausea during my pregnancies, I would take 1,000 milligrams of calcium and 500 milligrams of magnesium because the two work hand-in-hand.

Motion Sickness

I find that eating ginger is always great for stomach problems. I know this sounds like the wackiest thing I've written so far, but believe me it works! Tape an umeboshi plum (a Japanese salt plum) to your navel. It will cure all forms of motion sickness. Both of these can be found at your local health food store.

PMS

Five days before the onset of your period, avoid eating all extreme foods: nothing too sweet, nothing too salty, no alcohol. Limit your food to pastas, grains, vegetables, fruits, and light proteins. You will not believe how you sail through "those days."

Sprains

Grate some fresh ginger into a saucepan. Add vodka (don't use the good stuff) to cover, cook slowly. Do not eat. Put a dish towel over the sprain and the ginger/vodka mash on top of the towel over the sprained area. Do not put mash directly on the skin; it could cause a serious burn. Wrap aluminum foil around the outside of the towel to keep in the heat. Keep wrapped until mash cools.

20 | Practical Living in Your New Total Health Makeover World

*W*ell, you made it to the next-to-last chapter of the book. If you're like most people I have met, the information in these pages probably makes sense to you because it's logical (and it works). But one of the questions I hear over and over is "Marilu, how can I stay on this program in real life? I eat out at night, I have to feed my kids, I have business lunches all the time, and what if I'm invited to someone's home for dinner? Do I insult the host by asking him to leave the cheese off my potatoes au gratin?"

Well, good news! The information in these pages is realistic and simple to incorporate into your daily routine. You can easily (you'll be surprised at just how easily) overcome all these hurdles, gracefully and tactfully. Hey, we're talking about your health here!

How to Order in a Restaurant

The cool thing is that you order the same as you always did. You just eat differently. You will find that once you get the hang of food combining or eating a dairy-free diet, or any of the other steps, it's really pretty easy to order accordingly. I wanted to offer you the best possible advice on ordering in a restaurant to maintain your total health makeover so I went to someone I greatly admire for his expert advice. Louis Lanza, owner and chef of four restaurants in New York City (Josephina, Citrus Bar and Grill, The Blue Star, and my personal favorite, Josie's, a completely dairy-free restaurant) has taken the guesswork out of ordering for us. Who better to ask than an owner and chef of four of New York's (it's a tough town!) best restaurants?

❋   ❋   ❋   ❋   ❋   ❋   ❋   ❋   ❋   ❋

LOUIS LANZA
ON ORDERING IN A RESTAURANT:

If you're really getting into this seriously, and you want to stay on Marilu's program, I think the number one thing is to spend a few minutes and write down exactly what you *don't* want in your food. Make it as simple and easy to read as possible (no dairy, no meat, no sugar, etc.). And then have that list when you go into restaurants and give it to your service person. Most food servers, if you ask them whether something has dairy in it or if the soup stock is vegetarian, they say, "Yeah, yeah, yeah," and they might not even know. And half the time, they'll say, "There's no this, there's no that."

A lot of confusion occurs when it comes to being a vegetarian. Chefs use different stocks, like chicken stocks, or meat stocks. For example, when you ask for the roasted butternut squash soup, it could have chicken

257

stock in it. You could end up eating the things you didn't want. It's important to clarify with your waiter what you can and can't have. In my restaurants, the waiters have a full description of every single dish on the menu. There's a food manual, so they know exactly what the ingredients are in every dish. Write down what you can't eat, and what your substitutions are, and then give it to your food server, and say, "I'd appreciate it if you gave this to the chef." Even if you go to a place that isn't as health conscious as my restaurants, I think they'll respond better to your request if it's in writing. The chef's going to take a minute to look at it and say—okay. He knows what goes in the food. He's not going to serve you something on purpose that you don't want to eat. As long as this information gets back to the kitchen. Having something down on paper is better than having all these extremists who are vague about what they want come in saying, "I can't have this, I don't eat that." That's what causes confusion, because when you order, you're really talking to three different people. You're talking to a manager, your server, and by the time the chef gets the order, your order isn't happening the way you want it.

❋   ❋   ❋   ❋   ❋   ❋   ❋   ❋   ❋   ❋

Louis offers some great advice on ordering. Don't be ashamed of letting your server know that you have special needs. You wouldn't hesitate for a minute to ask if there are strawberries in the pie if you were deathly allergic to them, would you? That's how you have to think about ordering while following my program. A lot of people I know won't speak up in this kind of situation, but it's important to ask questions so you get what you want. Also, in researching restaurants for this book, I was happily surprised to find that almost every restaurant was only too happy to accommodate a "special" order.

I wanted to give you some samples from a couple of different restaurants to help you see how easy it can be. I have selected menus from a T.G.I.Friday's, Josie's, a Chinese restaurant, a deli, and an Italian restaurant.

❋　❋　❋　❋　❋　❋　❋　❋　❋　❋

THE FIVE EASY PIECES THEORY

At T.G.I.Friday's we have what is known as the Five Easy Pieces Theory. This theory stresses Friday's deep concern for our guests' satisfaction. We will go out of our way to honor a realistic guest request. Many of Friday's managers take a guest's request one step further, by getting the guest exactly what they want, even if the ingredients aren't in the restaurant.

Friday's Five Easy Pieces Theory was developed from the Jack Nicholson movie *Five Easy Pieces.* In the movie, Nicholson goes into a restaurant and orders a side of whole-wheat toast. The waitress made it clear that they did not serve whole-wheat bread. The annoyed waitress pointed to a sign in the restaurant that read "No Substitutions" and "We Reserve the Right to Refuse Service to Anyone." Nicholson ordered a chicken salad sandwich on whole-wheat toast, but told the waitress to hold the mayo, hold the lettuce, and hold the chicken salad and just bring him the whole-wheat toast. Unwisely, she asked where she should hold the chicken salad. On that note, he left as a very dissatisfied guest.

AMY FRESHWATER,
DIRECTOR OF PUBLIC RELATIONS
FOR FRIDAY'S HOSPITALITY WORLDWIDE, INC.

❋　❋　❋　❋　❋　❋　❋　❋　❋　❋

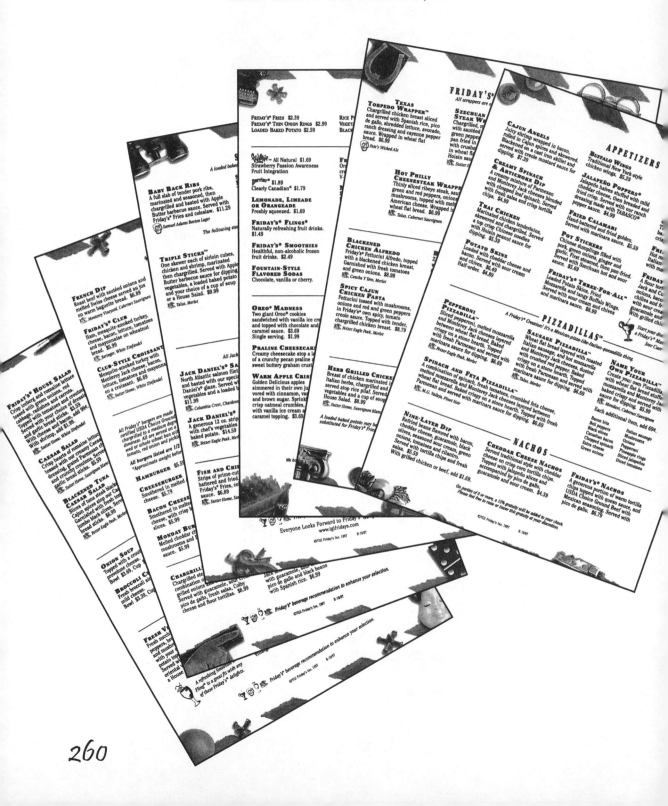

FRENCH DIP
Roast beef with sautéed onions and melted Swiss cheese served au jus on warm baguette bread. $6.89
Monterey Vineyard, Cabernet Sauvignon

FRIDAY'S CLUB
Ham, mesquite-smoked turkey, cheese, bacon, lettuce, tomatoes and mayonnaise on wheatnut bread. $5.99
Beringer, White Zinfandel

CLUB-STYLE CROISSANT
Mesquite-smoked turkey with Monterey Jack cheese, bacon, lettuce, tomatoes and mayonnaise on a croissant. $6.69
Sutter Home, White Zinfandel

BABY BACK RIBS
A full slab of tender pork ribs, marinated and seasoned, then chargrilled and basted with Apple Butter barbecue sauce. Served with Friday's Fries and coleslaw. $11.29
Samuel Adams Boston Lager

The following stea

TRIPLE STICKS™
One skewer each of sirloin cubes, chicken and shrimp, marinated then chargrilled. Served with Apple Butter barbecue sauce for dipping, vegetables, a loaded baked potato and your choice of a cup of soup or a House Salad. $9.99
Talus, Merlot

FRIDAY'S HOUSE SALAD
Crisp iceberg and romaine lettuce tossed with green onions, red cabbage, radishes and carrots. Topped with tomatoes and croutons. Served with your choice of dressing and garlic bread sticks. $2.59
With cheese and bacon, add 99¢
With shrimp, add $1.99.
Sutter Home, White Zinfandel

CAESAR SALAD
Crisp hearts of romaine lettuce tossed with our creamy Caesar dressing, grated Parmesan cheese and crunchy croutons. Served with garlic bread sticks. $5.69
Sutter Home, Sauvignon Blanc

BLACKENED TUNA
CAESAR SALAD
Slices of tuna steak blacke Cajun spices atop our Caesar Garnished with fresh tomat Jumbo black olives. Served bread sticks. $8.99
Fetzer Eagle Peak, Merlot

ONION SOUP
Topped with a crou provolone cheese.
Bowl $3.69, Cup

BROCCOLI C
Fresh broccoli
mild cheese.
Bowl $3.39, Cup

FRESH V
Fresh zucch
peppers, and
with your
potato to
Served w
oriental
s House

JACK DANIEL'S® SA
North Atlantic salmon filet and basted with our own Daniel's® glaze. Served w vegetables and a loaded b $11.99
Columbia Crest, Chardonn

JACK DANIEL'S®
A generous 12 oz. strip with chef's vegetables baked potato. $14.59
Fetzer Eagle Peak, Merl

FISH AND CHI
Strips of prime-cut battered and fried Friday's Fries, co sauce. $6.89

CHEESEBURGER
Smothered in melted cheese. $5.79

BACON CHEE
Smothered in crisp b slices. $5.99

MONDAY BUR
Melted cheddar c mushrooms and sauce. $5.99

CHARGRILL
Chargrilled ste combination w grilled onions Served with guacamole, sour pico de gallo, fresh salsa, Colby cheese and flour tortillas. $8.99

HAMBURGER $5.5

All Friday's burgers are made certified USDA Choice Ground chargrilled to a medium degree doneness. All are served on a seed or whole wheat bun ser tomato, red onion and pick

All burgers listed are 1/2
Approximate weight before

FRIDAY'S FRIES $2.39
FRIDAY'S THIN ONION RINGS $2.99
LOADED BAKED POTATO $2.59

A loaded baked

— All Natural $1.69
Strawberry Passion Awareness
Fruit Integration

perrier® $1.89
Clearly Canadian® $1.79

LEMONADE, LIMEADE
OR ORANGEADE
Freshly squeezed. $1.69

FRIDAY'S FLINGS®
Naturally refreshing fruit drinks. $1.49

FRIDAY'S SMOOTHIES
Healthful, non-alcoholic frozen fruit drinks. $2.49

FOUNTAIN-STYLE
FLAVORED SODAS
Chocolate, vanilla or cherry.

OREO® MADNESS
Two giant Oreo® cookies sandwiched with vanilla ice cre and topped with chocolate and caramel sauce. $3.69
Single serving. $1.99

PRALINE CHEESECAKE
Creamy cheesecake atop a l of a crunchy pecan praline sweet buttery graham crust

WARM APPLE CRIS
Golden Delicious apples simmered in their own ju vored with cinnamon, va and brown sugar. Sprink crisp oatmeal crumbles, with vanilla ice cream a caramel topping. $3.69

All Jack

RICE P
VEGETA
BLACK

FR
Or
cre
V

N
o
c

TEXAS
TORPEDO WRAPPER™
Chargrilled chicken breast sliced and served with Spanish rice, pico de gallo, shredded lettuce, avocado, ranch dressing and cayenne pepper sauce. Wrapped in wheat flat bread. $6.99
Pete's Wicked Ale

HOT PHILLY
CHEESESTEAK WRAPPE
Thinly sliced ribeye steak, sau green and red peppers, onions mushrooms, topped with melt American cheese. Wrapped in wheat flat bread. $6.99
Talus, Cabernet Sauvignon

BLACKENED
CHICKEN ALFREDO
Friday's Fettucini Alfredo, topped with a blackened chicken breast. Garnished with fresh tomatoes and green onions. $8.99
Concha Y Toro, Merlot

SPICY CAJUN
CHICKEN PASTA
Fettucini tossed with mushrooms, onions and red and green peppers in Friday's own spicy, tomato creole sauce. Topped with tender, chargrilled chicken breast. $8.79
Fetzer Eagle Peak, Merlot

HERB GRILLED CHICKEN
Breast of chicken marinated i Italian herbs, chargrilled and served atop rice pilaf. Served vegetables and a cup of soup House Salad. $8.99
Sutter Home, Sauvignon Blanc

A loaded baked potato may be substituted for Friday's Frie

FRIDAY'S
All wrappers are s

SZECHUAN
STEAK W
Chargrilled, m with sautéed green pepper fried in with crushe in wheat fla Hoisin sauc
Sutter H

FRIDAY'S
All wrappers are s

CAJUN ANGELS
Juicy shrimp wrapped in bacon, rolled in Cajun spices and skewered. Blackened on a cast iron skillet and served with creole mustard sauce for dipping. $7.39

CREAMY SPINACH
& ARTICHOKE DIP
A creamy mixture of Parmesan and Monterey Jack cheeses blended with chopped leaf spinach. Served with fresh salsa and crisp tortilla chips. $4.99

TRAI CHICKEN
Marinated chicken tenderloins, skewered and chargrilled. Served a top crisp Chinese noodles with Hoisin peanut sauce for dipping. $5.99

POTATO SKINS
Loaded with cheddar cheese and bacon. Served with sour cream and chives. $6.49
Half-order. $4.99

PEPPERONI
PIZZADILLA™
Sliced pepperoni, melted mozzarella and Monterey Jack cheese layered between wheat flat bread. Baked crispy on a stone hearth. Baked with fresh Parmesan and served with marinara sauce for dipping. $6.69
Fetzer Eagle Peak, Merlot

SPINACH AND FETA PIZZADILLA™
A combination of spinach, fresh tomatoes, melted mozzarella and Monterey Jack cheeses layered between wheat flat bread. Baked crispy on a stone hearth. Topped with fresh Parmesan and served with marinara sauce for dipping. $6.69
M.G. Vallejo, Pinot Noir

NINE-LAYER DIP
Refried beans flavored with bacon, cheddar cheese, guacamole, black olives, seasoned sour cream, green onions, tomatoes and cilantro. Served with tortilla chips and fresh salsa. $5.59
With grilled chicken or beef, add $1.69.

APPETIZERS

BUFFALO WINGS
Traditional New York-style chicken wings. $5.29

JALAPEÑO POPPERS®
Jalapeño halves stuffed with mild cheddar cheese, then batter and fried crisp. Served with our ranch dressing made with TABASCO® pepper sauce. $4.99

FRIED CALAMARI
Hand-battered and fried golden. Served with marinara sauce. $5.59

POT STICKERS
Chinese dumplings filled with pork, green onions, ginger and garlic. First steamed, then pan-fried. Served with Szechuan hot and sour sauce. $5.69

FRIDAY'S THREE-FOR-ALL™
Loaded Potato Skins, Fried Mozzarella and tangy Buffalo Wings. Served with sour cream and chives and marinara sauce. $6.99

PIZZADILLAS
A Friday's Creation! It's a Mexican-pizza-like-the-Italian-quesadilla thing.

SAUSAGE PIZZADILLA™
Wheat flat bread layered with Italian sausage, and hot mozzarella and Monterey Jack cheese, dusted with crumbled red pepper. Baked crispy on a stone hearth. Baked with fresh Parmesan and served with marinara sauce for dipping. $6.69
Mondavi, Cabernet Sauvignon

NAME YOUR
OWN PIZZADILLA™
Create your own Pizzadilla with wheat flat bread stuffed mozzarella and Monterey Jac sauce for dipping. $5.99
Each additional item, add 69¢.

Bacon bits   Italian sausage
Bell peppers   Onions
Black olives   Pepperoni
Canadian bacon   Pineapple rings
Chopped spinach   Sliced Jalapeño
Extra cheese   Diced tomatoes
Green onions

CHEDDAR CHEESE NACHOS
Served traditional style with cheddar cheese on crisp corn tortilla chips. Topped with jalapeño slices and accompanied by pico de gallo, guacamole and sour cream. $4.39

NACHOS

FRIDAY'S NACHOS
A generous portion of warm tortilla chips topped with queso sauce, and USDA Choice Ground Beef and Mexican seasoning. Served with pico de gallo. $6.79

FRI
Ho
on
Italian
chee
FRIDA

A flour tort
Jack and Co
onions, and
chiles and fr
guacamole a
With grilled c

Start your dini
a Friday's® Mar
Jose Cuer

On parties of 8 or more, a 15% gratuity will be added to your check.
Please feel free to raise or lower this gratuity at your discretion.

©TGI Friday's Inc. 1997   B-10/97

We h

Everyone Looks Forward to Friday's
©TGI Friday's Inc. 1997   B-10/97

©TGI Friday's Inc. 1997   B-10/97

Friday's® beverage recommendation to enhance your selection.

A refreshing Smoothie Fling® is a great fit with any of these Friday's® delights.

Friday's® beverage recommendation to enhance your selection.

T.G.I.Friday's

Appetizers:

✳ Potato skins. I'd skip the cheese and sour cream.

✳ Pizza. I'd order it with no cheese and all vegetables.

✳ Guacamole. I'd just have a little bit for my potato skins.

Salads:

✳ House Salad. Dressing on the side (vinaigrette or oil and vinegar).

✳ Blackened Tuna Caesar Salad. No cheese.

✳ Fresh Vegetable Medley. No cheese.

Main Dish:

✳ Veggie Wrapper. No cheese.

✳ Broken Noodles Pasta. No cheese.

✳ Jack Daniel's Salmon. No dairy.

✳ Pacific Coast Tuna. I'd skip the linguini and ask for steamed vegetables.

✳ Fish and Chips. Only if I'm in the mood for something really nasty and fattening and I'm not food combining that night.

Chinese Restaurant

✳ Cold Noodle and Sesame Sauce.

✳ Vegetable Steamed Dumplings.

✳ Moo Shoo Vegetables.

✳ Steamed Salmon in Black Bean Sauce.

✳ Dried Sautéed String Beans. No meat.

✳ Tofu with Three Different Nuts.

✳ *No MSG on anything!*

I could order so many items off this menu and still stay well within the boundaries of the ten steps.

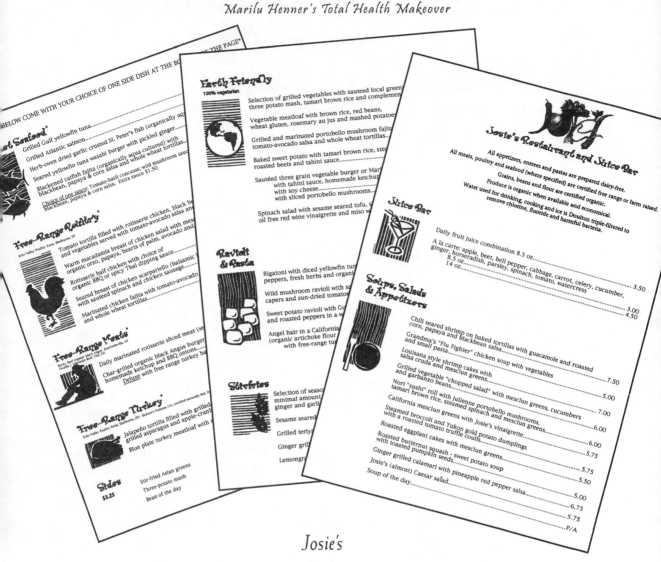

Josie's

❋ I'd eat anything except chicken or meat.

Deli

❋ Borscht. No sour cream.

❋ Lox, Egg Whites, and Onions. Cooked with oil or margarine.

❋ Bagel and Lox. I bring my own favorite tofu cream cheese.

❋ Tuna Fish Salad.

* Kasha.
* Smoked Sturgeon/Whitefish.
* Veggie Burger.

Italian Restaurant

* Grilled Portobello Mushrooms.
* Bruschetta.
* Arugula, Raddichio, and Tomato Salad.

Pasta

* Linguini Marinara.
* Fusilli with Broccoli and Garlic.
* Fusilli with Sundried Tomato and Broccoli.
* Pasta Primavera.

Entrees

* Grilled Fish of the Day (no butter).

Side Dishes

* Steamed or Sautéed Spinach.
* Broccoli with Garlic and Oil or Steamed.

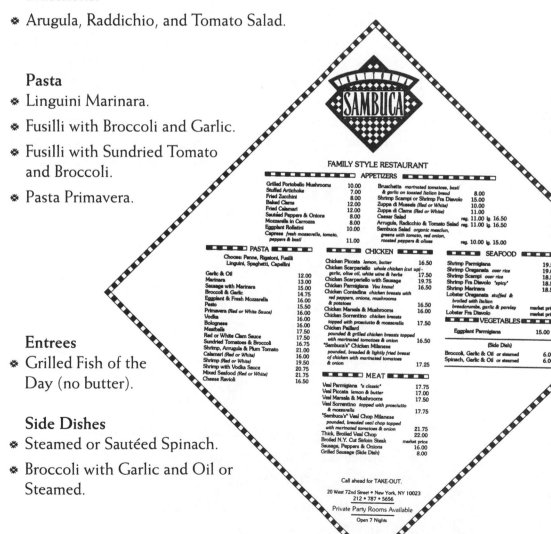

SAMBUCA

FAMILY STYLE RESTAURANT

APPETIZERS

Grilled Portobello Mushrooms	10.00	Bruschetta *marinated tomatoes, basil & garlic on toasted Italian bread*	8.00
Stuffed Artichoke	7.00	Shrimp Scampi or Shrimp Fra Diavolo	15.00
Fried Zucchini	8.00	Zuppa di Mussels *(Red or White)*	10.00
Baked Clams	12.00	Zuppa di Clams *(Red or White)*	11.00
Fried Calamari	12.00	Caesar Salad	reg. 11.00 lg. 16.50
Sautéed Peppers & Onions	8.00	Arrugula, Radicchio & Tomato Salad	reg. 11.00 lg. 16.50
Mozzarella in Carrozza	8.00	Sambuca Salad *organic mesclun,*	
Eggplant Rollatini	10.00	*greens with tomato, red onion,*	
Caprese *fresh mozzarella, tomato, peppers & basil*	11.00	*roasted peppers & olives*	reg. 10.00 lg. 15.00

PASTA

Choose: Penne, Rigatoni, Fusilli
Linguini, Spaghetti, Capellini

Garlic & Oil	12.00
Marinara	13.00
Sausage with Marinara	15.00
Broccoli & Garlic	14.75
Eggplant & Fresh Mozzarella	16.00
Pesto	15.50
Primavera *(Red or White Sauce)*	16.00
Vodka	16.00
Bolognese	16.00
Meatballs	17.50
Red or White Clam Sauce	17.50
Sundried Tomatoes & Broccoli	16.75
Shrimp, Arrugula & Plum Tomato	21.00
Calamari *(Red or White)*	16.00
Shrimp *(Red or White)*	19.50
Shrimp with Vodka Sauce	20.75
Mixed Seafood *(Red or White)*	21.75
Cheese Ravioli	16.50

CHICKEN

Chicken Piccata *lemon, butter*	16.50
Chicken Scarpariello *whole chicken (cut up) - garlic, olive oil, white wine & herbs*	17.50
Chicken Scarpariello with Sausage	19.75
Chicken Parmigiana *You know!*	16.50
Chicken Contadina *chicken breasts with red peppers, onions, mushrooms & potatoes*	16.50
Chicken Marsala & Mushrooms	16.00
Chicken Sorrentino *chicken breasts topped with prosciutto & mozzarella*	17.50
Chicken Paillard *pounded & grilled chicken breasts topped with marinated tomatoes & onion*	16.50
"Sambuca's" Chicken Milanese *pounded, breaded & lightly fried breast of chicken with marinated tomatoes & onion*	17.25

MEAT

Veal Parmigiana *"a classic"*	17.75
Veal Piccata *lemon & butter*	17.00
Veal Marsala & Mushrooms	17.50
Veal Sorrentino *topped with prosciutto & mozzarella*	17.75
"Sambuca's" Veal Chop Milanese *pounded, breaded veal chop topped with marinated tomatoes & onion*	21.75
Thick, Broiled Veal Chop	22.00
Broiled N.Y. Cut Sirloin Steak	market price
Sausage, Peppers & Onions	16.00
Grilled Sausage (Side Dish)	8.00

SEAFOOD

Shrimp Parmigiana	19.50
Shrimp Oreganata *over rice*	19.00
Shrimp Scampi *over rice*	18.50
Shrimp Fra Diavolo *"spicy"*	18.50
Shrimp Marinara	18.50
Lobster Oreganata *stuffed & broiled with Italian breadcrumbs, garlic & parsley*	market price
Lobster Fra Diavolo	market price

VEGETABLES

Eggplant Parmigiana	15.00
(Side Dish)	
Broccoli, Garlic & Oil *or steamed*	6.00
Spinach, Garlic & Oil *or steamed*	6.00

Call ahead for TAKE-OUT.

20 West 72nd Street • New York, NY 10023
212 • 787 • 5656
Private Party Rooms Available
Open 7 Nights

263

Stocking Your Pantry

Stocking up on all the essentials for your new life can be scary at first. Before you go out and shop for your new healthy replacements, you need to do a full sweep of your cupboards and refrigerator, and depending on which step or steps you're taking, get rid of any products that no longer work for your new lifestyle. (Don't throw out the nonperishable items. You can donate them to your local homeless shelter.)

I have made a shopping list for you to get started. Give yourself the opportunity to try healthy substitutes for the foods you've been eating that no longer work for your diet. You can get dairy-free puddings, pastries, soy cheese pizza. You name it and there's probably a substitute. (Remember that as you progress on this health makeover, your tastes are bound to change and foods you once craved might not be at the top of your list anymore.)

Breakfast Items

* Fruit juice-sweetened jams/jellies (Cascadian Farms, Sorrel Ridge).
* 100 percent flourless grain bread and cinnamon raisin bread (Ezekiel, Food for Life).
* Wheat-free breads (Baldwin Hill, Windmill Farms).
* Nondairy rice, soy, and almond milk (Imagine Foods Rice Dream, Westbrae, Pacific).
* Nondairy cream cheese.
* Egg whites from a free-range or "certified organic" farm.
* Fresh-squeezed juices.
* Soy yogurt (White Wave).
* Cereals (Erewhon, Nature's Path, Barbara's).
* Breakfast sausages (Soy Boy).

Lunch and Dinner Items

❋ Soups (Hain Pure Foods, Health Valley).

❋ Chicken and turkey products—hot dogs, sausages, and patties (Shelton's).

❋ Meat substitutes—Canadian bacon, pepperoni, tofu dogs (Yves).

❋ Ravioli with soy cheese (Soy Boy).

❋ Veggie burgers, tofu lasagna, soy cheese and macaroni (Amy's).

❋ Frozen dairy-free Italian dinners (Legume).

❋ Vegan burger patties (Boca Burger).

❋ Frozen chicken patties and nuggets, veggie munchies, pizza munchies (Health Is Wealth).

❋ Lentil rice loaf, okara patties (Natural Touch).

Snacks

❋ Rice cakes (Hain Pure Foods, Lundberg).

❋ Rice crackers (Edward and Sons, San J).

❋ Pretzels, peanut butter pretzels, potato sticks.

❋ Veggie sticks (Natural GH).

❋ Hummus. A variety of flavors is available, and you can use this as a replacement for cheese (Abraham's, Cedar).

❋ Bean dips (Guiltless Gourmet).

Americans average 22 percent of calories a day from snack foods. It's 7 percent in France.

❋ Nut butters—peanut, cashew, almond, etc. (Maranatha Natural Foods).

❋ Potato chips (Poppers, Rubert's, Garden of Eatin, Westbrae, Kettle Chips).

* Fruit juice-sweetened cookies (Frookies, Health Valley, Barbara's, Hain Pure Foods).
* Healthy salsa (Enricos Organic, Garden Valley Naturals).
* Ice creams (Imagine Foods Rice Dream Ice Cream, Ice Bean, Sweet Nothings).
* Puddings (Imagine Foods).
* Organic applesauce with infused fruits (Solano Gold, Santa Cruz).

Cheese Substitutes

* Veggie singles (Light n' Less by Soyco).
* Rice and soy cheeses, including grated Parmesan (Light n' Less by Soyco).

Condiments

* Sea salts (Natural Sea).
* Organic miso (American Miso).
* Soft and firm tofu (Nasoya).
* Tofu sour cream.
* Nayonnaise (Nasoya).
* Organic fruit juice-sweetened ketchup (Westbrae, Muir Glenn, Shedds).
* Mustard (Tree of Life, Westbrae).
* Relishes (Cascadian Farm).
* Soybean margarine (Willow Run, Shedds).
* Salad dressings (Nasoya Foods).
* Soy sauce replacement (Dr. Bronner's, Bernard Jensen's).
* Liquid amino acids-soy sauce replacement (Braggs).

❋ Maple syrup, fruit juice syrup, rice syrup, barley malt (Shady Maple Farms).

❋ Succanat organic dried and milled sugar.

Drinks

❋ Fruit juice spritzers (R.W. Knudsen).

❋   ❋   ❋   ❋   ❋   ❋   ❋   ❋   ❋   ❋

LOUIS LANZA ON STOCKING UP

If I were to guide someone into a grocery store, looking for some substitute dairy products, one of the things I would do is get them to choose good quality products.

There are probably ten tofu sour creams out there, but there are only a few good ones. You have to go for quality. See what tastes better to you. Your taste buds have to be happy. Snacks used to be tough. It was so easy to grab some Ritz crackers and some cheddar cheese and start eating that. But now there are so many great healthy snacks out there. It's so much more accessible to us. There are veggie sticks, that are kind of like potato chips, only made out of potatoes and carrots. There are puddings and ice cream made from soybeans. It's not Häagen-Dazs, but it's a lot better than frozen yogurt. It tastes a lot richer than most low-fat or fat-free ice cream. You're going to be really surprised. And don't be fooled by fat-free products, either. All fat-free means is twice as many carbohydrates, so watch out for these. You don't have to be in a big city to find healthy options. Health food stores are all over the place. But a lot of these products can be found in grocery stores all over the country, too. Don't give up on these products if you try something or a particular brand and you don't like it. Think of it like dating. You have to kiss a lot of frogs before you meet your princess. (Or prince.)

❋　　❋　　❋　　❋　　❋　　❋　　❋　　❋　　❋　　❋

When thinking of a health food store, a lot of people get this vision of "granola head" hippies walking around in sandals and love beads shouting, "Make love, not war." Times have changed dramatically since those days. In fact, many cities have gourmet health markets that have replaced those hippie-dippie health food stores (although those stores still very much exist). These modern markets carry fresh and organic produce and free-range meats, poultry, and fish. Their selection of products rivals that of a larger chain food store. Most regular chain food stores have an organic foods section these days, too. Even in a city like New York (where a large grocery store is hard to find) you can find specialty stores that offer a variety of healthy snacks and fresh produce. You might have a good time exploring these stores. You never know. You just might like what you find.

Eating at a Friend's Home

This is always a sticky situation. I have made it easier by calling my friends in advance of the dinner and simply explaining to them my restrictions. Of course, most of my friends already know I don't eat dairy so it's usually not a problem. But I also don't eat meat, sugar, anything with chemicals, caffeine, and well, you know the rest of the list from this book. Most of the time it's not a problem. I never expect someone to change a menu based on what my dietary restrictions are, so I adapt to what they're serving. I might eat a salad and whatever vegetable is being served. That usually gets me through a tough spot. But lately, quite frankly, I have found that more people are eating the way I do, or at least a little closer to some variation of my diet, so it's become much easier and less intrusive on my part. Besides, I often find that people are curious about the way I eat, so this is usually a good opportunity for me to spread the word about this program. (I've met some of my best friends this way!) I will sometimes call ahead to *gently* remind my host or hostess of my eating restrictions, and every single time the call is appreciated. If you are eating at the home of good friends, they will definitely understand. If it's a business dinner or a dinner with someone you don't know well, keep in mind that most people are cooking healthier these days, so you ought to be able to make something work. One trick I've learned over the years, if I really think there's going to be *nothing* for me to eat, is to eat ahead of time. At the dinner, take a piece of bread or something else that you can eat, and break it up on your plate. Take small samplings of other foods, so that your plate doesn't look empty. Push it around with your fork so that the food looks touched. (Sometimes, faking is better!)

Flying

Airplane food has come a long way, so flying is no excuse to fall off the program. I order a dairy-free vegetarian meal in advance whenever I fly. My entire family eats the same meals, and depending on the airline, sometimes they're really quite good. I'll always bring my own snacks on a flight, too. The kids like to snack, and on long trips, I'm glad I have a little something along for myself!

Marilu Henner 101

Things I Have Learned About Health

1. Your health is the single most important factor of your life.
2. Remember that dis-ease is nothing more than lack of health.
3. He who can not find time for health will have to find time for illness.
4. Degenerative diseases come from behavior that departs from what our evolutionary past has adapted us to.
5. It's never too late to feel better than you do right now.
6. Listen to your body.
7. Your body is always looking for balance.
8. It's been my experience that the people most out of balance, when given the right information tend to be the most natural healers.
9. There's nothing better for facing a problem than a good night's sleep.
10. Sleep brings the answers.
11. Health is a state of mind.
12. Your mind is the boss.
13. A person is as old as his arteries.
14. Like cures like.
15. Floaters are better than sinkers.

Things I Have Learned About Food

16. Food is not an enemy, but a powerful friend.
17. Let food be your medicine and medicine be your food.
18. If you improve the quality of your food, the quantity takes care of itself.
19. Your stomach doesn't have teeth.
20. Don't eat your next meal until you feel resolved from your last meal.

21. Eat only one concentrated food per meal.
22. Try to let twelve hours pass once a day between concentrated food meals, i.e. dinner to breakfast.
23. Eat only when you're hungry.
24. Centered food creates centered behavior.
25. Fruits clean, vegetables build.
26. The fresher the pick the better.
27. Dine when you eat.
28. Taste what you're eating.
29. Man has the same teeth and intestines as grain eaters.
30. Flesh eaters sweat through their tongues.
31. Read what you're eating.
32. If you can't pronounce it, why in the world would you put it in your body?
33. You don't have to drink milk to make milk.

Beauty Tips

34. Before you even get out of bed, while your muscles are warm, do a light stretch.
35. Brush your teeth for one full minute.
36. Skin brush for two minutes every day to sweat evenly all over your body.
37. Break a sweat at least ten minutes every day.
38. Put a thin coat of Vaseline on your feet before putting on your workout socks.
39. Wear two pairs of socks and two exercise bras when doing anything aerobic.
40. In winter the best way to take care of your skin is to exfoliate, exfoliate, exfoliate.
41. Use an ice cube to tighten pores after washing your face.
42. Pin your pantyhose to the back of your bra for a long, roll-free look.

Things I Have Learned from Macrobiotics

43. All things are part of one infinity.
44. Everything changes.
45. All antagonisms are complementary.
46. There is nothing identical.
47. Whatever has a front has a back.
48. The bigger the front the bigger the back.
49. Whatever has a beginning has an end.

Things I Have Learned from My Parents

50. People should be blamed for their sicknesses, not pitied.
51. Anything that suggests an accident is an accident.
52. A little bit of chemistry, a little bit of physics.
53. Always have a spare.
54. Put on a little lipstick.

Things My Therapist Says

55. Have all your feelings, but use judgment when putting them into action.
56. Depression is anger turned inward.
57. A guilty parent is the worst parent.
58. Sometimes crying is tears of rage.
59. Your reputation is everything.
60. If you treat something like it's an emergency, and it isn't, you get into trouble.

Things My Life Has Taught Me

61. The key to your life is how well you deal with plan B.
62. You only feel old if you're not where you want to be, and you don't feel you have the time to get there.
63. Attitude is everything.
64. Ask yourself, "Is it worth the headache?"

65. "Is it worth the stomachache?"
66. "Is it worth the heartache?"
67. When in doubt, throw it out.
68. Better a bad announcement than a bad marriage.
69. Give any problem, argument, drama, thirty-six hours and watch it change.
70. In trying to make a decision, pretend to make one choice. Live with it for a few hours, and see how you feel. Make the other choice, do the same. See which feels better.
71. If you can't decide what to do, do nothing.
72. Have a good laugh at least once a day.
73. Have a good cry at least once a week.
74. Be a good friend; practice friend maintenance.
75. If you feel bad about something, don't throw a pity party, do something nice for someone else.
76. You can usually tell a lot about a person by how you feel about yourself after you've been with them.
77. Everything after eighth grade is a repeat.
78. You're never afraid to face a situation if you've done your homework.
79. Sometimes you have to go through bad to get to good.
80. Everything is connected to everything.
81. The magic is in the mix.
82. God is in the details.
83. Never look back unless you're planning to go that way.
84. The best way to get out of a difficulty, is to get through it.
85. The truth you usually don't have to make a lot of noise about.
86. Sometimes, laughter is the laughter of recognition.
87. You lose your power when you yell.
88. Sometimes, faking is better.
89. Know what you're getting yourself into and you'll know where you're going.
90. Life can be easy. It's how much stuff you put in your way that makes it your life.
91. Confucius say: Why do you hurt me? I haven't helped you!

92. When you're really nervous, your sense of humor and your sexuality go out the window.
93. The more I want to get something done, the less I call it work.
94. By all means, keep on moving.

Things I Say to My Kids

95. Shake it off.
96. Cut the drama.
97. 10 yards for bad acting.

Things My Kids Say

98. Mommy says "no screaming, no biting, no dairy products, no sugar."
99. "But I'm not tired!"
100. "You the Poo Poo Man!"

B.E.S.T. ADVICE:

101. WORK THE COAT!

21 | Some Final Thoughts

*W*hen I sat down to write this book, I really had enough information in my head to fill the pages of three books! I wanted to share everything I have learned over the past nineteen years and help you get on the road to health and happiness. I've only skimmed the surface of my information pool in this book, but I hope that you have some new things to consider about your life.

I received a lot of feedback from friends and family who had the unique opportunity to read advance copies of this book. What I found so fascinating is how many people said they've been wanting to change, at the very least, one thing on my list. They just didn't know how. Friends thanked me for opening their thought processes and helping them to regain control over their lives. Health is not just the opposite of disease, it is a way of life.

I know that I've thrown a lot of information at you at once. Don't become overwhelmed by the seemingly daunting task ahead of you. Take it *one step* and *one day* at a time.

Change is never easy, but you can face the challenge that lies ahead because you are so much better equipped with this new-found knowledge and information. Don't get discouraged if you try and don't succeed at first. Failure is only failure if you never try.

I hope you'll find yourself talking about what you read in my book to loved ones. I want you to become a conduit of information, just as I have. Passing this information along will strengthen your conviction about the importance of maintaining your new healthy life. And better yet, you will improve the quality and quantity of your time on this planet.

Every now and then, something comes along and taps us on the shoulder as a little reminder that we must take care of our bodies, and ourselves. There's no such thing as an accident, and you do in fact have control over your journey. You have choices in life, no matter who you are. As I said earlier in this book, health isn't everything, but without it, you've got nothing.

Take care and be well!

Marilu

Appendix A: Rich Sources of Nutrients

ANTIOXIDANTS

Vitamin E
Vitamin C
Selenium
Coenzyme Q 10
L-carnosine
L-methionine
L-taurine
L-glutathione
Polyphenols
Phytochemicals
Ascorbyl palmitate
Vitamin B12
Pantothenic acid
Thiamine
Riboflavin
Niacin
Folic acid
Zinc citrate
Inositol
Copper
Beta-carotene

ANTIOXIDANT FOODS

Yams
Butternut and winter
   squash
Pumpkin
Carrots
Spinach
Broccoli
Iceberg lettuce
Endive
Kale
Tomatoes
Cantaloupe
Apricots
Mango
Papaya

VITAMIN A

Eggs
Yellow fruits and
   vegetables
Fish-liver oil

VITAMIN B1

(thiamine)
Brewer's yeast
Whole grains
Wheat germ
Whole-grain flour
Rice bran
Blackstrap molasses

VITAMIN B1 *(continued)*
Brown rice
Fish and poultry
Salmon
Egg yolks
Legumes
Chickpeas
Kidney beans
Navy beans
Soybeans
Sunflower seeds

VITAMIN B2
(riboflavin)
Fish
Eggs
Almonds
Chicken
Brewer's yeast
Wheat germ

VITAMIN B3
(niacin)
Beets
Brewer's yeast
Turkey
Chicken
Fish
Salmon
Swordfish
Tuna
Sunflower seeds
Peanuts

VITAMIN B6
(pyridoxine)
Avocados
Bananas
Carrots
Lentils
Brown rice
Bran
Soybeans
Sunflower seeds
Filberts
Tuna
Shrimp
Salmon
Wheat germ
Whole-grain flour

VITAMIN B12
(cyanocobalamin)
Eggs
Fish
Clams

BIOFLAVONOIDS
Citrus fruits
Fruits
Black currants
Buckwheat

BIOTIN
Egg yolks
Liver
Unpolished rice

BIOTIN (continued)
Brewer's yeast
Whole grains
Sardines
Legumes

VITAMIN C
Citrus fruits
Rose hips
Acerola cherries
Alfalfa seeds,
   sprouted
Black currants
Guava
Papaya
Grapefruit
Lemons
Orange juice
Tomatoes
Pimientos
Cantaloupe
Strawberries
Kiwi fruit
Broccoli
Tomatoes
Red sweet peppers
Green peppers
Brussels sprouts
Broccoli
Cabbage
Cauliflower
Kale
Peas

CALCIUM
Green leafy vegetables
Collards
Broccoli
Tofu
Soybeans
Okra
Shellfish
Mackerel
Salmon
Sardines
Molasses
Bone meal
Dolomite

CHLORINE
Table salt
Seafood
Ripe olives
Rye flour
Dulse

CHROMIUM
Honey
Grapes
Raisins
Corn oil
Clams
Whole-grain cereals
Brewer's yeast

COENZYME Q10
Spinach

COENZYME Q10 (continued)

Peanuts

Tuna

Sardines

COPPER

Wheat germ

Barley

Lentils

Brazil nuts

Cashews

Filberts

Peanuts

Oatmeal

Molasses

VITAMIN D

Eel

Pilchard

Salmon

Sardines

Herring

Mackerel

Tuna

Vitamin-D fortified
    soy milk

Egg yolks

Fish-liver oils

Bone meal

VITAMIN E

Cold-pressed oils

Eggs

Wheat germ

Molasses

Sweet potatoes

Leafy vegetables

Sunflower seeds

Walnuts

Peanuts

Brazil nuts

Cashews

Pecans

Almonds

Hazelnuts

Wheat germ

Soybeans

Lima beans

FLUORIDE

Tea

Seafood

Fluoridated water

Bone meal

FOLIC ACID

Spinach

Asparagus

Turnip greens

Brussels sprouts

Lima beans

Soybeans

Chicken liver

Brewer's yeast

Root vegetables

Whole grains

Wheat germ

Bulgur wheat

FOLIC ACID (continued)

Kidney beans

White beans

Oysters

Salmon

Orange juice

Avocado

IODINE

Seafood

Kelp

Iodized salt

IRON

Eggs

Fish and poultry

Blackstrap molasses

Cherry juice

Green leafy
   vegetables

Dried fruits

VITAMIN K

Green leafy
   vegetables

Egg yolks

Safflower oil

Blackstrap molasses

Cauliflower

Soybeans

MAGNESIUM

Seafood

Whole grains

Dark green vegetables

Molasses

Nuts

Bone meal

NIACIN

Poultry and fish

Brewer's yeast

Peanuts

Rice bran

**PANTOTHENIC ACID
(vitamin B5)**

Brewer's yeast

Corn

Lentils

Egg yolks

Peas

Peanuts

Soybeans

Sunflower seeds

Whole-grain flower

Lobster

Whole grains

Wheat germ

Salmon

PHYTOCHEMICALS

Soybeans and soy
   products

Hot chili peppers

Tomatoes

Broccoli

Citrus fruits

Berries

PHYTOCHEMICALS (continued)

Apricots

Garlic

Onions

POTASSIUM

Red snapper

Salmon

Whole grains

Potatoes

Beet greens

Acorn squash

Avocado

Apricots

Bananas

Cantaloupe

Tomato juice

Orange juice

Peaches

Prunes

Soybeans

Lima beans

Swiss chard

Yams

Spinach

Dried fruits

Blackstrap molasses

Sunflower seeds

SELENIUM

Tuna

Herring

Oysters

Clams

Brewer's yeast

Wheat germ and bran

Whole grains

Wheat flour

Puffed wheat

Sesame seeds

Brazil nuts

Sunflower seeds

SODIUM

Seafood

Table salt

Baking powder

Baking soda

Celery

Kelp

UNSATURATED FATTY ACIDS

Vegetable oils

Sunflower seeds

ZINC

Pumpkin seeds

Squash seeds

Sunflower seeds

Seafood

Oysters (the highest)

Crabmeat

Herring

Mushrooms

Brewer's yeast

Soybeans

Eggs

Wheat germ

Turkey

Appendix B:
Josie's Recipes

MISO BROTH WITH VEGETABLES
SERVINGS: 2

16 oz. filtered water
3 shiitake mushrooms, cleaned and sliced
3 cremini mushrooms, cleaned and sliced
2 oz. carrots, julienne
2 oz. bok choy (asparagus can be substituted)
2 oz. firm tofu ½" disc
2 scallions sliced thin
1 1" x 6" sheet toasted nori (seaweed)
1 tbsp. organic miso or to taste

- Heat water in small pot.
- Add vegetables and simmer for 2–3 minutes.
- Pour into bowl over tofu.
- Stir in miso*.
- Garnish with sliced scallion and toasted nori julienne.

* *Never put Miso into boiling water. Remove from stove before mixing.*

Nutritional Analysis Per Serving: 79 Calories, 2 g Total Fat, 0 mg Cholesterol, 343 mg Sodium, 12 g Carbohydrate, 5 g Protein

BUTTERNUT SQUASH SOUP
SERVINGS: 6

$\frac{1}{2}$ tbsp. chopped shallot
$\frac{1}{2}$ tbsp. chopped garlic
$\frac{1}{2}$ cup diced $\frac{1}{4}$" leeks
$\frac{1}{2}$ cup diced $\frac{1}{4}$" yellow onion
$\frac{1}{8}$ tsp. dry oregano
$\frac{1}{8}$ tsp. dry thyme
$\frac{1}{8}$ tsp. dry basil
3 drops Tabasco
$\frac{1}{8}$ tsp. celery salt
$1\frac{1}{2}$ tsp. sea salt
1 lb. peeled diced $\frac{1}{4}$" sweet potato
3 cups filtered water
$1\frac{1}{2}$–2 cups soy milk
1 medium butternut squash (no skin) halved, seeded, roasted
1 tbsp. honey
$\frac{1}{2}$ tsp. cinnamon
$\frac{1}{2}$ tsp. nutmeg
3 tbsp. pumpkin seeds (toasted)

- Sauté the shallot, garlic, leeks, yellow onion, oregano, thyme, basil, Tabasco, celery salt, and sea salt together for 5 minutes or until onions are tender.
- Add diced sweet potato and water and let boil until sweet potato is tender.
- Add cooked squash with its juice.
- Simmer for 15 minutes over medium heat, add milk, and puree mixture.
- Season to taste.
- Butternut squash to be cooked by roasting in the oven for 40–50 minutes at 500°, seasoned with honey, cinnamon, nutmeg, and 1 cup filtered water, cover with foil.
- Garnish with toasted pumpkin seeds.

Nutritional Analysis Per Serving: 219 Calories, 4 g Total Fat, 0 mg Cholesterol, 1,827 mg Sodium, 43 g Carbohydrate, 6 g Protein

BLACK BEAN DUMPLINGS

SERVINGS: *4 servings of 3 dumplings each*
YIELD: *12 dumplings*

1 cup cooked black beans (mashed)
¼ cup tahini (ground sesame seed)
1 oz. scallion, chopped fine
1 tbsp. tamari
1 tbsp. mirin
½ tsp. rice wine vinegar
½ tsp. ponzu (Japanese citrus)
salt and ground pepper to taste
1 tbsp. chili garlic paste
12 dumpling skins (available at Asian markets)

- Mix all ingredients together in bowl except for dumpling skins.
- Put water around the dumpling skin.
- Add 1 tsp. of black bean stuffing, seal tight.
- Sauté in nonstick pan rubbed with olive oil.
- Brown 1 minute on each side. Finish in 350° oven 3 minutes.

Nutritional Analysis Per Serving: 247 Calories, 10 g Total Fat, 2 mg Cholesterol, 391 mg Sodium, 27 g Carbohydrate, 11 g Protein

ORGANIC RED MISO DIP WITH MANGO
Sauce for Black Bean Dumplings

SERVINGS: 4

1 tbsp. organic red miso
2 oz. filtered water
2 tbsp. mirin
1 tbsp. ponzu
1 tbsp. chive
2 tbsp. diced mango

- Whisk first 4 ingredients together. Add mango and chive.

Nutritional Analysis Per Serving: 19 Calories, 0 g Total Fat, 0 mg Cholesterol, 157 mg Sodium, 3 g Carbohydrate, 1 g Protein

CHILI-SEARED SHRIMP MARINADE
Marinade for 3 dozen medium shrimp

YIELD: *36 shrimp*
SERVINGS: *9 servings of 4 shrimp each*

36 medium shrimp, peeled and cleaned
1½ tsp. ground coriander seed
2 oz. tomato paste
1½ oz. tamari
1 oz. mirin
2 tbsp. chili garlic paste
1 tbsp. lemon juice
1 tbsp. olive oil
1½ tbsp. ancho chili powder (mild chili can be substituted for any chili powder)

- Whisk all ingredients together.
- Add shrimp, refrigerate a minimum of 6 hours, up to 26 hours.
- Sear in hot nonstick pan rubbed with olive oil, one minute on each side.
- Serve on baked tortilla chips with a dollop of guacamole and seared shrimp set on top.

Nutritional Analysis Per Serving: 141 Calories, 6 g Total Fat, 95 mg Cholesterol, 851 mg Sodium, 7 g Carbohydrate, 15 g Protein

GUACAMOLE
for Chili-Seared Shrimp

SERVINGS: 8

2 avocados
$\frac{1}{2}$ cup diced $\frac{1}{4}$" red onion
$\frac{1}{2}$ cup diced tomato (no seeds)
1 tbsp. chopped cilantro
$\frac{1}{4}$ tsp. Tabasco
$\frac{1}{4}$ tsp. hot sauce
$\frac{1}{8}$ tsp. cayenne pepper powder
$\frac{1}{2}$ tsp. lemon juice
salt and pepper to taste

- Mash all ingredients together, season with salt and pepper.

Nutritional Analysis Per Serving: 77 Calories, 8 g Total Fat, 0 mg Cholesterol, 7 mg Sodium, 2 g Carbohydrate, 1 g Protein

CHOPPED VEGETABLE SALAD

2 beefsteak tomatoes, sliced thick
1 bunch asparagus, ends cleaned
1 large green bell pepper, top and bottom sliced off
2 ears corn on the cob, shucked
3 large carrots, peeled and sliced thick lengthwise
1/4 lb. fresh green beans, ends trimmed
10 cloves garlic, minced
1/3 cup Dijon mustard
3/4 cup olive oil
1 head Romaine lettuce, washed and sliced thin

- In a large bowl add garlic and 2 ounces of olive oil. Add all vegetables except lettuce, season with salt and fresh ground black pepper. Grill vegetables on medium heat and set aside.
- Chop all vegetables into medium size pieces. Just before serving, add vinaigrette, and place on top of shredded romaine lettuce.

VINAIGRETTE

- Mix balsamic vinegar and Dijon mustard in bowl and slowly add remaining 4 oz. of olive oil while whisking.

Nutritional Analysis Per Serving: 258 Calories, 18 g Total Fat, 0 mg Cholesterol, 85 mg Sodium, 22 g Carbohydrate, 5 g Protein

ORGANIC ARTICHOKE FLOUR PASTA WITH ORGANIC PLUM TOMATO SAUCE

YIELD: *approx. 6 servings of sauce*

2 tbsp. extra-virgin olive oil
5 cloves sliced garlic
3 oz. yellow onion diced small
12 basil leaves rolled and sliced thin (chiffonade)
1½ tbsp. tomato paste
32 oz. can organic plum tomatoes, sliced
½ tsp. red chili flakes
2 tsp. salt
3 oz. (dry weight) organic artichoke flour angel hair pasta

- Heat oil in a skillet and sauté garlic and onions until lightly browned.
- Add half the basil and the tomato paste.
- Continue to cook for 2 more minutes.
- Add drained tomatoes (sliced lengthwise) to pan.
- Simmer 10–12 minutes and add salt and chili flakes.
- Cook angel hair pasta in boiling salted water until half done and drain.
- Add pasta to sauce and cook on low flame until some of the sauce has been absorbed into the pasta.
- Transfer to a serving bowl, sprinkle the remaining basil on top and, and serve.

Nutritional Analysis Per Serving: 349 Calories, 6 g Total Fat, 0 mg Cholesterol, 1,067 mg Sodium, 63 g Carbohydrate, 11 g Protein

SUPER SOY CAESAR

¹⁄₄ cup soy parmesan
2 small cloves of garlic
¹⁄₃ cup olive oil
1 tsp. of worcestershire
1 tsp. Dijon mustard
Juice of ¹⁄₂ lemon
4–6 fillets of anchovies
1 egg yolk
3 heads Romaine lettuce, washed and cut into large pieces.
Non-dairy croutons (optional)

- Mix egg yolk, garlic, worcestershire, mustard, lemon juice, and anchovies in food processor, slowly drizzle in the olive oil. Season with salt and fresh ground pepper.
- In a large mixing bowl toss Romaine lettuce with dressing, sprinkle in soy parmesan and fresh ground black pepper. Serve with croutons if desired.

Nutritional Analysis Per Serving: 89 Calories, 5 g Total Fat, 58 mg Cholesterol, 408 mg Sodium, 6 g Carbohydrate, 9 g Protein

TURKEY TORTILLA ROLL
2 SERVINGS

1 tsp. garlic
1 tsp. each of oregano, thyme, and sage, mixed
$\frac{1}{8}$ tsp. each of sea salt and pepper, mixed
8 oz. turkey breast (pound thin)
4 oz. julienne mixed vegetables (carrot, zucchini, yellow squash, and red cabbage)
1 tsp. olive oil
$\frac{1}{2}$ tsp. garlic
sea salt and pepper to taste
apple-cranberry chutney (see following recipe)
10" flour tortilla

- Marinate the turkey breast with the garlic, oregano, thyme, and sage for a minimum of one hour, then grill or sauté.
- Sauté mixed vegetables with garlic in olive oil, season with salt and pepper, and let cool.
- Put cranberry chutney 2 tbsp. around flour tortilla
- Arrange cooled julienne vegetables in the center of the tortilla.
- Add grilled turkey breast sliced $\frac{1}{4}$" thick on top of vegetables.
- Season with a touch of salt and pepper, roll up the tortilla.
- Heat in microwave for 40 seconds.
- Serve with your favorite bean dish for good food combining.

Nutritional Analysis Per Serving: 287 Calories, 9 g Total Fat, 88 mg Cholesterol, 629 mg Sodium, 45 g Carbohydrate, 46 g Protein

APPLE-CRANBERRY CHUTNEY
Garnish for Turkey Tortilla Roll

SERVINGS: *8 2 oz. servings*

1 tbsp. brandy
$1/4$ cup rice wine vinegar
1 cup orange juice
$1/2$ tsp. minced ginger
2 cups cranberries (fresh or frozen)
$1/2$ cup diced $1/4$ yellow onions
2 oz. fruit juice sweetener
$1/4$ tsp. sea salt

- Deglaze the brandy.
- Add rice wine vinegar, orange juice, and minced ginger and simmer for 20 minutes.
- Add frozen cranberries and simmer until tender.
- Add diced onions and fruit juice sweetener and simmer for 20 minutes.
- Season with salt.

Nutritional Analysis Per Serving: 67 Calories, 0 g Total Fat, 0 mg Cholesterol, 74 mg Sodium, 15 g Carbohydrate, 0 g Protein

STIR FRY SAUCE
SERVINGS: *4–6 (4 oz. per serving)*
YIELD: *3¾ cups*

½ cup sherry or Marsala wine
3 oz. fresh ginger, sliced
1 tbsp. shallots, chopped
1 tbsp. garlic, chopped
1 cup mirin
3/4 cup wheat-free tamari
2 cups filtered water
2 tbsp. arrow root powder (mixed with 2 tbsp. filtered water)
toasted sesame seeds (optional)

- Deglaze sherry/Marsala wine with ginger, shallots, and garlic by half.
- Add mirin, tamari, and filtered water, let boil for 5 minutes.
- Add arrow root powdered mix and simmer for 5 minutes.
- Sauté 1½ cups of your favorite seasonal vegetables in 4 oz. of Stir Fry Sauce.
- Serve with 4 oz. of brown rice, season with salt and pepper.
- Sprinkle with toasted sesame seeds if desired.

Nutritional Analysis Per Serving: 96 Calories, 0 g Total Fat, 0 mg Cholesterol, 2,015 mg Sodium, 9 g Carbohydrate, 4 g Protein

TERIYAKI SAUCE
SERVINGS: 8

2 cups filtered water
2 oz. ponzu (Japanese citrus)
2½ oz. tamari
6 oz. fruit juice sweetener
1 tbsp. arrow root powder (mixed with 1 tbsp. filtered
  water)

- Mix all ingredients (except arrow root powder).
- Allow to boil for 10 minutes.
- Add arrow root powder, boil for 5 more minutes.
- Brush on chicken/vegetables or fish while sautéing or broiling.
- Serve with stir-fry vegetables.

Nutritional Analysis Per Serving: 95 Calories, 0 g Total Fat, 0 mg Cholesterol, 495 mg Sodium, 23 g Carbohydrate, 1 g Protein

VEGETARIAN MEAT LOAF
SERVINGS: 8

$\frac{1}{2}$ tsp. garlic
$\frac{1}{2}$ tsp. shallots
1 cup yellow onions (fine diced)
1 cup carrots (fine diced)
1 cup corn kernels
1 cup celery (fine diced)
$\frac{1}{2}$ cup mixed bell peppers (fine diced)
$\frac{1}{4}$ tsp. dried thyme
$\frac{1}{4}$ tsp. dried oregano
$\frac{1}{2}$ tsp. dried basil
1 oz. wheat-free tamari
1 oz. mirin
$\frac{1}{2}$ tsp. ground black pepper
2 cups cooked lentils
2 cups plain brown rice
$\frac{1}{2}$ cooked kabocha squash
1 tsp. salt
2 cups fresh ground bread crumbs

- Mix 1 tbsp. canola oil, sauté garlic, shallot, onion, peppers, carrot, corn, and celery.
- Add tamari, mirin, and dry herbs.
- Cook approximately 15 minutes until vegetables are tender.
- In large mixing bowl add cooked brown rice, cooked lentils, and cooked kabocha squash.
- Fold in vegetables, season with salt and pepper, mix in fresh ground bread crumbs thoroughly.
- Mold into 9" Pyrex loaf pan.
- Bake at 350° for 30 minutes, let cool, and slice into 1" slices.

Nutritional Analysis Per Serving: 203 Calories, 2 g Total Fat, 0 mg Cholesterol, 581 mg Sodium, 40 g Carbohydrate, 9 g Protein

SWEET POTATO—RED MISO GRAVY
Sauce for Vegetarian Meat Loaf

SERVINGS: 8 *(4 oz. each)*

1 qt. water
2 cups diced ½" sweet potato
1 cup diced onion
½ tsp. sea salt
pinch ground pepper
2 oz. red miso

- Bring water to a boil.
- Add 1½ cups of sweet potato, ½ cup of onion, salt, and pepper.
- Simmer 20 minutes.
- Puree.
- Add ½ cup of sweet potato and ½ cup yellow onions.
- Remove from stove.
- Mix in miso.
- Serve under slice of Vegetarian Meat Loaf.

Nutritional Analysis Per Serving: 108 Calories, 1 g Total Fat, 0 mg Cholesterol, 415 mg Sodium, 24 g Carbohydrate, 2 g Protein

PORTOBELLO MUSHROOM FAJITA

1 jumbo portobello mushroom, steamed (2 medium can be
   substituted)
3 slices Bermuda onion sliced thin
5 slices red bell pepper sliced thin crosswise
5 slices yellow bell pepper sliced thin crosswise
2 tsp. extra-virgin olive oil
1 tbsp. balsamic vinegar
salt to taste
fresh ground black pepper to taste
2 8" whole-wheat tortillas

- Rub both sides of mushroom with balsamic vinegar, olive oil, salt, and pepper.
- Grill or broil both sides until mushroom feels tender in the center.
- Season peppers and onions with remaining balsamic vinegar and olive oil.
- Grill or broil until soft.
- Slice mushroom, lay on plate with peppers and onions on top.
- Serve with soft flour tortillas, your favorite salsa, and the sour cream.

Nutritional Analysis Per Serving: 306 Calories, 10 g Total Fat, 0 mg Cholesterol, 374 mg Sodium, 46 g Carbohydrate, 9 g Protein

CILANTRO TOFU SOUR CREAM
Garnish for Portobello Mushroom Fajita

8 oz. firm tofu
$\frac{1}{4}$ cup chopped cilantro
1 tsp. sea salt
$\frac{1}{2}$ cup filtered water
2 tbsp. lemon juice

- Puree all ingredients together, season with salt.

Nutritional Analysis Per Serving: 18 Calories, 1 g Total Fat, 0 mg Cholesterol, 302 mg Sodium, 1 g Carbohydrate, 2 g Protein

PICO DE GALLO
Salsa for Portobello Mushroom Fajita

YIELD: *4 servings*

1 cup plum tomatoes, diced small
2 tbsp. red onions, diced small
2 tsp. cilantro, chopped
1 tsp. jalapeño, seeded and finely diced
1 tbsp. olive oil
salt and pepper to taste

- Mix all ingredients in a bowl.

BANANA HONEY SPICE CAKE
(dairy & sugar free)

YIELD: *3 ten" layers*

4–5 ripe bananas
1 cup sucanat (available in health-food stores)
1 cup honey
1 cup canola oil
3 large eggs, separated
1 tbsp. vanilla extract
1 cup hot water
1 cup walnuts, chopped
3 cups whole-wheat pastry flour
$2^{1}/_{4}$ tsp. baking soda
$^{1}/_{2}$ tsp. salt
1 tbsp. cinnamon

- Preheat the oven to 350°. Spray 3 10" cake pans.
- With an electric mixer, cream the banana, sucanat, honey, and canola oil. Add the egg yolks and the vanilla.
- In a large bowl, combine the dry ingredients and add to the banana mixture alternately with the water, beginning and ending with the dry ingredients.
- Beat the egg whites stiff, but not dry, and fold them into the batter.
- Pour the batter into the prepared pans, smooth the top, and bake for 30 minutes or until the cake begins to pull away from the sides of the pan and a tester inserted in the center of the cake comes out clean. Cool on a wire rack and frost with Honey Meringue Frosting (see following recipe).

Nutritional Analysis Per Serving: 482 Calories, 11 g Total Fat, 35 mg Cholesterol, 405 mg Sodium, 96 g Carbohydrate, 7 g Protein

HONEY MERINGUE FROSTING

1 cup honey
2 large egg whites, room temperature
¼ tsp. salt
1 tsp. vanilla extract

- In a small saucepan on the stove or in a measuring cup in the microwave, bring the honey to a boil.
- In a mixing bowl beat the egg whites until stiff, add the salt, and slowly drizzle in the boiling honey in a steady stream. Beat continuously for several minutes until the frosting thickens.
- Add the vanilla and continue beating until the frosting becomes very thick. Use immediately or store in the refrigerator for later use. Frosts 3 10" layers.

HEALTHIER BISCOTTI
YIELD: *approximately 4 dozen biscotti*

$4\frac{1}{2}$ cups organic unbleached white flour
1 tsp. salt
2 tsp. baking powder
2 cups sucanat (available in health-food stores)
3 tsp. egg replacer (egg whites can be substituted)
6 oz. Wesson vegetable oil
3 tsp. vanilla extract
$1\frac{1}{2}$ cups chopped almond or walnuts

- Sift flour, salt, and baking powder.
- Beat sucanat, egg replacer, and vegetable oil.
- Add sifted mixture to beaten mixture.
- Add vanilla and chopped almonds or walnuts to mixture.
- Roll into logs 3" wide (approximately 4 logs).
- Bake 30 minutes at 350°.
- Cool 1 hour and slice into $\frac{3}{4}$" cookies.
- Bake on side 8–10 minutes.
- Store in airtight container.

Nutritional Analysis Per Serving: 128 Calories, 5 g Total Fat, 0 mg Cholesterol, 66 mg Sodium, 18 g Carbohydrate, 2 g Protein

HEALTHIER PUMPKIN PIE
(dairy & sugar free)

1 tsp. cinnamon
$\frac{1}{2}$ tsp. ginger
$\frac{1}{2}$ tsp. nutmeg
$\frac{2}{3}$ cup sucanat (available in health-food stores)
3 large eggs, lightly beaten, free-range
1 cup vanilla-flavored soy milk
2 cups pumpkin puree*
1 pie shell, unbaked

- Preheat the oven to 350°.
- In a large bowl, whisk together the spices and sucanat to remove any lumps. Whisk in the eggs, vanilla-flavored soy milk, and the pumpkin.
- Pour into an unbaked crust and bake until set, 50–60 minutes.

* *You may use fresh pumpkin or canned pumpkin. To use fresh, peel, cut up, and boil a small pumpkin until tender, and then puree in a food processor or blender. To use canned pumpkin, use 1 small can (15 oz.) organic pumpkin puree.*

Nutritional Analysis Per Serving: 206 Calories, 8 g Total Fat, 80 mg Cholesterol, 141 mg Sodium, 30 g Carbohydrate, 4 g Protein

HEALTHIER PIE CRUST
YIELD: *one 9" pie crust*

$^1/_4$ cup Arrowhead Mills oat flour
1 cup Arrowhead Mills spelt flour
$^1/_8$ tsp. sea salt
1 tbsp. sucanat
2 tbsp. tofu, soft
2 tbsp. soy margarine
3 oz. water, filtered cold

- Mix all the dry ingredients in a food processor on pulse for 1 minute. Add the soy margarine and tofu and mix for 2 minutes. Add the cold water and mix for an additional 1 minute.
- Remove from food processor and form into a ball. Roll out to approximately 10 inches and form in a 9-inch pie pan. It can be frozen at this point if you cover it with plastic wrap, or proceed to the next step of prepping.

MACADAMIA APPLE PIE
YIELD: *8 servings*

1 recipe Healthier Pie Crust
7 whole apples, Granny Smith
2 tbsp. sucanat
2 tsp. cinnamon, ground
1 tbsp. Arrowhead Mills spelt flour

¾ cup Arrowhead Mills spelt flour
¾ cup oats, rolled (raw)
6 tbsp. sucanat
⅛ tsp. sea salt
¼ cup macadamia nuts
¼ cup applesauce
¼ cup soy margarine

- Roll out pie dough into 9-inch round pan. Set aside.
- Filling: Thinly slice the peeled apples and toss them in a bowl with 2 T. sucanat, 2 t. cinnamon, and 1 T. spelt flour.
- Topping: Mix thoroughly the ¾ cup spelt flour with the oats, 6 tbsp. sucanat, sea salt, macadamia nuts, applesauce, and ¼ cup soy margarine.
- Put the apples into the uncooked pie shell and layer the rolled oat topping over the filling. Bake in preheated 300° oven for 1 hour.
- Serve warm with vanilla soy ice cream.

Nutritional Analysis Per Serving: 386 Calories, 15 g Total Fat (36.4% of calories from fat), 12 mg Cholesterol, 201 mg Sodium, 55 g Carbohydrate, 4.6 g Protein

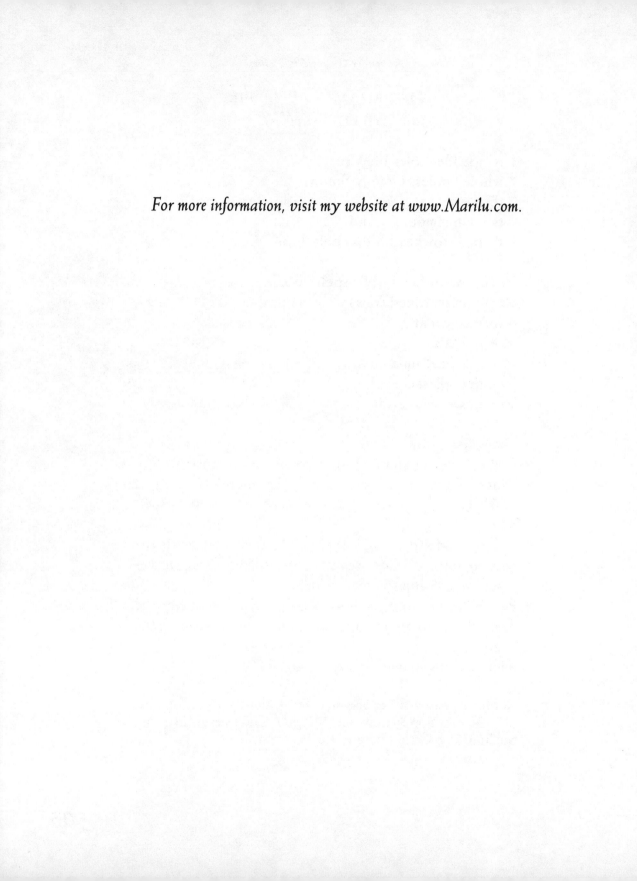

For more information, visit my website at www.Marilu.com.

Bibliography

Adato, Allison. "Living Legacy: Is Heredity Destiny?" *Life* (1997): 60–69.

Arnot, Robert. *Dr. Bob Arnot's Guide to Turning Back the Clock*. New York: Little, Brown and Co., 1995.

Baker, Sidney MacDonald. *Detoxification & Healing: The Key to Optimal Health*. New Canaan, Conn.: Keats Publishing, 1997.

Barnard, Neal. *Food for Life: How the New Four Food Groups Can Save Your Life*. New York: Crown Trade Paperbacks, 1993.

Beling, Stephanie. *Power Foods*. New York: HarperCollins Publishers Inc., 1997.

Bethel, May. *The Healing Power of Natural Foods*. North Hollywood: Wilshire Book Co., 1978.

Brody, Jane E. *The New York Times Book of Health: How to Feel Fitter, Eat Better and Live Longer*. New York: Random House, 1997.

Carey, Benedict. "The Talking Cure for Stress." *Health* (November/December 1996): 69–74.

Cassileth, Barrie R. *The Alternative Medicine Handbook*. New York: W.W. Norton & Co., 1998.

Cheney, Susan Jane. "Macrobiotics Demystified." *Vegetarian Times* (April 1994).

Christiano, Donna. "When Stress Goes to Your Stomach." *Good Housekeeping* (May 1997): 78, 81.

Cohen, Robert. *Milk: The Deadly Poison*. Englewood Cliffs, N.J.: Argus Publishing, 1997.

Davis, Susan. "Why We Must Sleep?" *American Health* (April 1996): 76–78.

Diamond, Harvey, and Marilyn Diamond. *Fit for Life*. New York: Warner Books, 1985.

Dufty, William. *Sugar Blues*. New York: Warner Books, 1975.

Faelten, Sharon, ed. *Food and You*. Emmaus, Pa.: Rodale Press, 1996.

Finch, Steven. "To See Your Future Look into Your Past." *Health* (October 1996): 93–94, 98–100.

Foltz-Gray, Dorothy. "Seven Herbs to Stock Up On—And Keep You Out of the Doctor's Office." *Prevention* (November 1997): 97–103.

Foreyt, John P., and G. Ken Goodrick. *Living Without Dieting: A Revolutionary Guide for Everyone Who Wants to Lose Weight*. New York: Warner Books, 1992.

Gallo, Nick. "Alternative Medicine: Is It for You?" *Better Homes and Gardens* (May 1995).

Gray, Robert. *The Colon Health Handbook*. Oakland, Calif.: Rockridge Publishing Co., 1983.

Houck, Catherine. "When Stress Gets Under Your Skin." *Good Housekeeping* (May 1996): 52–55.

Jensen, Bernard. *Dealing with the Reversal Process and the Healing Crisis Through Eliminating Diets and Detoxification*. Provo, Utah: BiWorld Publishers, 1976.

———. *Foods That Heal*. Garden City Park, N.Y.: Avery Publishing Group, 1993.

———. *Nature Has a Remedy*. Escondido, Calif.: Bernard Jensen, 1978.

———. *A New Lifestyle for Health & Happiness*. Escondido, Calif.: Bernard Jensen Enterprises, 1980.

Jensen, Bernard, and Mark Anderson. *Empty Harvest*. Garden City Park, N.Y.: Avery Publishing Group, 1990.

Jibrin, Janis. "Sweet It Is." *American Health* (December 1995): 59–61.

Kirschmann, Gayle J., and John D. Kirschmann. *Nutrition Almanac*. New York: McGraw Hill, 1996.

Klaper, Michael. *Pregnancy, Children and the Vegan Diet*. Maui, Hawaii: Gentle World, 1987.

Kushi, Michio. *Natural Healing Through Macrobiotics*. Tokyo: Japan Publications, 1978.

———. *Oriental Diagnosis: What Your Face Reveals*. London: Sunwheel Publications, 1981.

Kushi, Michio, and Aveline Kushi. *Raising Healthy Kids*. Garden City Park, N.Y.: Avery Publishing Group, 1994.

Leff, Michael, ed. "No More Meat?" *Consumer Reports on Health* (October 1995): 109–112.

Mason, Michael. "The Man Who Has a Beef with Your Diet." *Health* (May/June 1994): 53–58.

Michaud, Ellen, and Lila Anastas. *Listen to Your Body: A Head-to-Toe Guide to More Than 400 Symptoms, Their Causes and Best Treatments.* New York: MJF Book, 1998.

Michaud, Ellen, and Elisabeth Torg. *Total Health for Women.* Emmaus, Pa.: Rodale Press, 1995.

Miller, Saul. *Food for Thought: A New Look at Food & Behavior.* Englewood Cliffs, N.J.: Prentice-Hall, 1979.

Mindell, Earl. *Secret Remedies: The Essential Guide to Treating Common Ailments with Vitamins, Minerals, Herbs and Other Cutting-Edge Supplements.* New York: Fireside, 1997.

Napier, Kristine. "Green Revolution: Cancer-Fighting Foods." *Harvard Health Letter* (April 1995).

National Institute of Diabetes and Digestive and Kidney Diseases. "Your Digestive System and How It Works." National Digestive Diseases Information Clearinghouse: 1992.

Paulsen, Barbara. "A Nation Out of Balance." *Health* (October 1994): 45–48.

Pitchford, Paul. *Healing with Whole Foods.* Berkeley, Calif.: North Atlantic Books, 1993.

Prevention Magazine, ed. *Everyday Health Tips.* 1988.

Puhn, Adele. *The Five Day Miracle Diet.* New York: Ballantine Books, 1996.

Rampton, Sheldon, and John Stauber. *Mad Cow USA.* Monroe, ME.: Common Courage Press, 1997.

Tennesen, Michael. "Good Fat, Bad Fat." *Living Fit* (August 1997): 75–79, 116.

Thompson, W. Grant. *Gut Reactions: Understanding Symptoms of the Digestive Tract.* New York: Plenum Press, 1989.

Time-Life Books. *The Alternative Advisor: The Complete Guide to Natural Therapies and Alternative Treatments.* New York: Time-Life Books, 1997.

Vogel, Shawna. "Good Mood Foods." *Health* (October 1996): 71–74.

Walker, N.W. *The Natural Way to Vibrant Health*. Phoenix, Az.: O'Sullivan Woodside & Co., 1983.

Weinhouse, Beth. "Eleven Health Questions to Ask Your Mother Now." *Glamour* (April 1997): 85–93.

Weiss, Rick. "What's the Matter with Milk?" *Health* (January/February 1993): 18–20.

"What Can Caffeine Do for You and to You." *Consumer Reports on Health* (September 1997): 97, 99–101.

Index

Accent, 51
Acesulfame K
  dangers of, 49
  description of, 72
Acid-forming foods, and examples
  of B.E.S.T. foods, 34
Acid indigestion, 227
Acupressure, 245, 249
Acupuncture, 245, 248–249
Additives. *See also* Chemicals
  (B.E.S.T. step 1)
  children's diet and, 48
  dangers of, 49–55
  FDA definition of, 47
  reasons for using, 46–48
Adrenaline, 240
Airplane food, 269
Alcohol
  food combining and, 116, 117
  heartburn and, 227
  irritable bowel disease and, 224
  reading your face and, 202, 203
Alkaline-forming foods, and
  examples of B.E.S.T. foods, 34
Allergies
  food, 238–241
  milk, 88, 97, 98
Alternative medicine, 245–255
  acupuncture and, 248–249
  Eastern and Western medicine
    and, 247–248
  herbal supplements and, 251–253
  homeopathic medicine and,
    249–251
  qi and balance in, 245–246
  secret cure-alls and, 253–255

shiatsu and acupressure and, 249
Aluminum, and detoxification, 41
American Dietetic Association, 72,
  82
American Heart Association, 123
American Medical Association, 172
Amino acids, and carbohydrates, 32
Ana-Kit, 240
Anaphylaxis, and food allergies,
  239–240
Animal foods, and yin and yang,
  22–24
Anorexia, 175
Antacids, and heartburn, 227
Antibiotics, in milk, 89
Antioxidants
  skin care and, 208
  sources of, 277
  usefulness of, 252–253
  vegetarian diet and, 83
Appetite suppressant medications,
  180
Apple-cranberry chutney, recipe for,
  293
Aqua Buzz, 58
Arthritis, and dairy use, 84, 88
Artichoke flour pasta with organic
  plum tomato sauce, organic,
  recipe for, 290
Artificial colorings. *See also* Additives
  dangers of, 49–50
Artificial sweeteners. *See* Sugar
  substitutes *and specific products*
Aspartame
  dangers of, 50–51
  description of, 72

Aspirin, and heartburn, 227
Attention Deficit Disorder, and
  sugar use, 77
Attention Deficit Hyperactive
  Disorder, and sugar use, 77
Ayurvedic medicine, 246

Bacteria
  diarrhea and, 222
  E. coli contamination and, 57
  inflammatory bowel disease and,
    225
  slaughterhouse methods and, 82
  stool content and, 217
  sugar use and oral, 76
Balance, 19–35
  centering your body and, 33–35
  changing your palate and, 27–29
  description of yin and yang in,
    19–22
  diet and, 24–26
  examples of nutritional foods in,
    34
  extreme foods and, 22–24
  food and behavior and, 26–27
  qi in alternative medicine and,
    245–246
Banana honey spice cake, recipe for,
  300
Barley malt, 73
Baths, 142–144
Beauty tips, 271
Beinfeld, Harriet, 247
Belching, 219–220
Bergson, Henri, 245
B.E.S.T., 3–4

description of, 15–16
excuses for not following, 12–13
making the commitment to start, 36–39
ten steps of, 4–9
as a workable program, 10–12
BHA (butylated hydroxyanisole), 51
BHT (butylated hydroxytoluene), 51
Biotin, 278–279
Birth control pills, 226
Biscotti, healthier recipe for, 302
Black bean dumplings, recipe for, 285
Blindness, and synthetic fats, 53
Blood pressure
    caffeine and, 60, 63–64
    fiber and, 230
    genetics and, 191
    vegetarian diet and, 83
Body
    balancing/centering of, 33–35
    benefits of calcium for, 91–92
    caffeine use and, 58–59, 63–64
    dairy use and, 84, 85
    detoxification and healing crises and, 40–43
    ideal weight and, 183
    laughter and, 140
    listening to signals from, 232–244
    need for sleep and, 149–150
    skin brushing and, 144–146
    stress and, 135
    sugar use and, 76–77
Body image
    dieting and, 176
    questions to think about, 15
Body weight. *See* Weight
Bones
    caffeine use and, 64
    milk and, 87
    osteoporosis and, 195–198
    vegetarian diet and, 83
Borstelmann, Jim, 100
Bowel movements, 209–232
    digestive system and, 210–212
    effort involved in, 216–217

frequency of elimination and, 213
    lifestyle journal recording, 213, 235, 242
    stool consistency in, 215–216
    stool weight in, 214–215
    transit time in, 215
Brain, and sleep, 151–152
Bran, 229
Breakfast, stocking your pantry for, 264
Breast cancer
    dairy and, 95
    fiber and, 229, 230
    genetics of, 195
Breast feeding, 96–97
Brown, Rita Mae, 37
Brown sugar, 71
Bulimia, 175
Butter, alternatives to, 103
Butternut squash soup, recipe for, 284–285
Butylated hydroxyanisole (BHA), 51
Butylated hydroxytoluene (BHT), 51

Caesar salad, super soy recipe for, 291
Caffeine (B.E.S.T. step 2), 5, 58–64
    benefits of, 60–61
    chemical structure of, 59
    dependency on, 61–62
    detoxification and, 41
    diarrhea and, 222, 223
    food allergies and, 239
    health risks of, 63–64
    irritable bowel disease and, 224
    jet lag and, 254
    makeover tips for wimps, 45
    overload in diet of, 60
    pregnancy and, 64
    side effects of using, 58–59
    stimulation from, 58–59
    stress and, 141
    withdrawal symptoms from, 61
Caine, Michael, 10–11, 116
Cake, banana honey spice, recipe for, 300
Calcium
    benefits of, 91–92

caffeine use and, 64
    constipation from, 220
    food combining and, 115, 117
    in foods, 89–91
    milk and, 87, 93
    morning sickness and, 254
    osteoporosis and, 196, 197–198
    skin care and, 208
    sleep and, 156
    sources of, 279
    as a supplement, 251
    vegetarian diet and, 83
Calories
    eating habits and, 169
    exercise and, 131–133
    fat and, 124
    milk and, 93
    sugar and, 68, 77
Campylobacter, 82
Cancer
    artificial colorings and, 50
    acesulfame K and, 72
    butylated hydroxyanisole (BHA) and butylated hydroxytoluene (BHT) and, 51
    dairy and, 95–96
    fat and, 123
    fiber and, 228, 230
    genetics of, 195
    rBGH (recombinant bovine growth hormone) and, 54
    saccharin and, 54, 71
    synthetic fats and, 53
Candy
    constipation and, 220
    gas and, 219
    heartburn and, 227, 228
    skin problems and, 204
Cane juice, 74
Carbohydrates
    diarrhea and, 223
    examples of B.E.S.T. foods in, 34
    inflammatory bowel disease and, 226
    milk and, 93, 95
    no-fat diets and, 179
    as a nutritional category, 32
    stress and, 141

Carbonated beverages
  caffeine in, 58, 59, 62
  gas and, 219
Carney, JoAnn, 44
Centers for Disease Control, 57, 222
Chanel, Coco, 205
Cheese
  alternatives to, 102
  food allergies and, 239
  problems from eating, 85
  substitutes for, 266
Chemical additives. *See* Additives
Chemical preservatives. *See* Preservatives
Chemicals (B.E.S.T. step 1), 4, 46–57
  dangers of, 49–55
  detoxification and, 41
  FDA definition of additive and, 47
  makeover tips for wimps, 45
  organic food certification and, 55–57
  reasons for using, 46–48
  smoking and, 65
Chewing, 29–30
Chicken, slaughterhouse methods for, 80–81
Children
  aspartame and, 51, 72
  balance in diet and, 25–26
  breast feeding and, 96–97
  chemical additives and, 48
  eating habits developed by, 174–176
  Marilu Henner 101 on, 274
  milk and allergies in, 88, 97
  nitrites and, 53
  sugar use and, 67–68
Chili-seared shrimp marinade, recipe for, 289
Chinese food, 51–52
Chinese medicine, 245, 246
  acupuncture and, 248–249
Chinese restaurant, ordering from, 261
Chlorine, 82, 279
Chocolate

caffeine in, 59, 62
food allergies and, 239
heartburn and, 227, 228
irritable bowel disease and, 224
mood and, 234
Cholesterol
  fat and, 120, 122–124
  fiber and, 228, 229
  milk and, 86–87
  vegetarian diet and, 83
Chopped vegetable salad, recipe for, 289
Chromium, 279
Chutney, apple-cranberry, recipe for, 293
Cilantro tofu sour cream, recipe for, 299
Clinical depression, 193–194
Cocoa bean, 62
Coenzyme Q10, 279–280
Colas, caffeine in, 62
Colds, cure for, 253–254
Cold sores, cure for, 253
Colitis, 224
Collagen, 204–205, 208
Colon
  digestion and, 212
  irritable bowel disease (IBS) and, 224–225
  stool content and blood in, 217
Colon cancer, and fiber, 230
Color additives, 48
Complexion
  moisturizers and, 206–207
  stress and, 207
  sun and, 205
  vitamins and minerals for helping, 207–209
Condiments, stocking your pantry for, 266–267
Confidence, 164–165
Constipation, 220–222
  bowel movement effort and, 216
  causes of, 220–221
  fiber and, 229
  stool consistency and, 215
  tips for avoiding, 221–222
Copper, 280

Crohn's disease, 226

Dairy (B.E.S.T. step 5), 6, 84–104
  alternatives to, 101–104
  breast feeding and, 96–97
  cancer and, 95–96
  comments on experiences of giving up, 99–101
  detoxification and, 41
  diarrhea and, 223
  fat and, 98–101
  food allergies and, 238
  gas and, 219
  heart disease and, 192
  how cows are treated and, 85–87
  makeover tips for wimps, 45
  nutrient deficiencies and, 96
  rBGH (recombinant bovine growth hormone) and, 54, 94–95
  reading your face and eating, 202, 203
Davidson, Michael H., 229
Deli, ordering from, 262–263
Depression, 193–194
Detoxification, 40–43
  healing crises and, 41–43
  need for, 40–41
  two-step process of, 41
Diabetes
  fiber and, 230
  genetics and, 198–199
  sugar use and, 76
Diamond, Harvey and Marilyn, 108
Diarrhea, 222–223
  bowel movement effort and, 216
  causes of, 222
  food allergies and, 239
  inflammatory bowel disease and, 226
  irritable bowel disease and, 224
  recovery from, 222–223
  stool consistency and, 215
Diary. *See* Journal
Diet. *See also* Food; Food combining (B.E.S.T. step 6)
  additives in. *See* Additives
  balance in, 24–26

behavior and, 26–27
cancer and, 195
changing your palate and, 27–29
chewing and, 29–30
children and, 25–26
constipation and, 220–222
diarrhea and, 222–223
eating at a friend's home,
    268–269
fiber in, 228–231
five tips on, 30–31
gas and, 219–220
herbal supplements and, 251–252
identifying what is right in,
    38–39
limiting fat in, 124–126
making the commitment to
    change, 36–39
no-fat diets and, 178–180
nutritional categories in, 31–33
opposites attract in, 25
ordering in a restaurant, 257–263
personal hygiene and, 27
preservatives in. *See* Preservatives
quitting smoking and, 66
reading your face and, 201–204
skin problems and, 204
stocking your pantry, 264–268
stress reduction and, 247
unhealthy lifestyle of Americans
    and 1–3
weight and, 169
yin and yang and extremes in,
    22–24
Dieting, 168–184
    balancing/centering your body
        and, 35
    being healthy and, 171
    differences between men and
        women in, 174–178
    fad diets and, 172–173
    fat cells and, 125
    ideal weight and, 183
    no-fat diets and, 178–180
    questions to think about, 14–15
    set point and, 184
Digestion

chewing and, 29–30
dairy use and, 85
disorders of, 217–228
fat and, 125
food combining and, 107–109
mechanism of, 210–212
reading your face and, 202
sugar and, 69
Dinner, stocking your pantry for,
    265
Dopamine, and stress, 141
Drescher, Fran, 10, 85, 98–99
Drugs
    caffeine use and, 62
    constipation from, 220
    dieting and, 172–173, 180–181
    sleep problems and, 154
Dyes in food, dangers of, 49–50

Eastern medicine, 245, 246–247. *See
    also* Alternative medicine
Eating. *See* Food; Food combining
    (B.E.S.T. step 6)
Echinacea, 254
E. coli, 57
Eden Soy, 101
Eggs, alternatives to, 102–103
Elimination. *See* Bowel movements
Energy, and fat, 120–121
Epinephrine, 240
EpiPen, 240
Equal, 50, 72
Exercise and stress (B.E.S.T. step 8),
    7–8, 127–146
    baths and, 142–144
    calories and, 131–133
    Eastern medicine and, 247
    effects of stress, 135
    laughter and, 140
    lifestyle journal recording, 235,
        241
    makeover tips for wimps, 45
    osteoporosis and, 198
    reasons for stress, 134
    reducing stress, 136–145
    right level of exercise in, 128–129
    skin brushing and, 144–146

target heart rate and, 129
Exfoliation, 206
Exitotoxin, 52

Face
    reading, 200–208
    skin brushing and, 146
Fajita, portobello mushroom, recipe
    for, 298
Family Health History Chart, 186,
    188–189
Fat (B.E.S.T. step 7), 7, 119–126
    cholesterol and, 122–124
    constipation from, 220
    dairy and, 98–101
    examples of B.E.S.T. foods in, 34
    food combining and, 116
    heartburn and, 227
    heart disease and, 192
    irritable bowel disease and, 224
    limiting, 124–126
    makeover tips for wimps, 45
    meat and, 80
    milk and, 86, 93
    no-fat diets and, 178–180
    as a nutritional category, 33
    overview of, 120–121
    quiz on, 119–120
    synthetic fats and, 53–54
    types of, 121–122
Fat-free foods
    diets with, 178–180
    stocking your pantry, 267–268
FDA. *See* Food and Drug
    Administration
Fiber, 228–231
    amount of, in common foods,
        230–231
    constipation and lack of, 220
    food allergies and, 239
    inflammatory bowel disease and,
        226
    irritable bowel disease and, 225
    reasons for eating, 229–230
    stool weight and, 214
Fight or flight response, 135, 193
Five Easy Pieces Theory, 259

Flatley, Michael, 175
Fluoride, 280
Fluoride toothpaste, 76
Flying, 269
Folic acid
  pregnancy and, 251
  sources of, 280–281
Food
  additives in. *See* Additives
  allergies to, 238–241
  balance in diet and, 24–26
  behavior and, 26–27
  changing your palate and, 27–29
  chewing and, 29–30
  children and, 25–26
  constipation and, 220–222
  cravings for, 233–234
  diarrhea and, 222–223
  eating at a friend's home,
    268–269
  eliminating pesticides by washing,
    57
  fiber in, 230–231
  five tips on, 30–31
  gusto and, 165–166
  herbal supplements and, 251–252
  intolerances to, 238–241
  lifestyle journal recording, 235, 237
  Marilu Henner 101 on, 270–271
  nutritional categories in, 31–33
  opposites attract in, 25
  ordering in a restaurant, 257–263
  personal hygiene and, 27
  preservatives in. *See* Preservatives
  questions to think about, 13–14
  reading your face and, 201–202
  skin problems and, 204
  stocking your pantry, 264–268
  stress and, 141
  yin and yang and extremes in,
    22–24
Food additives. *See* Additives
Food allergies, 238–241
  anaphylaxis and, 239–240
  causes of, 238
  lifestyle journal on, 241
  milk and, 88, 97, 98

  symptoms of, 238–239
Food labels. *See* Labels
Food preservatives. *See* Preservatives
Food and Drug Administration
  (FDA)
  additives approved by, 47
  artificial colorings and, 49
  aspartame and, 50, 72
  bacteria and *E. coli* and, 57
  fat blockers and, 181
  sulfites and, 55
  synthetic fat and, 53
Food combining (B.E.S.T. step 6),
  6–7, 105–118
  basic idea of, 105–106
  charts on, 112–113
  "fix it" chart for, 118
  guidelines for, 110–111
  how it works, 107–110
  makeover tips for wimps, 45
  reasons for using, 106–107
  stress and, 141–142
  tips on, 113–117
Food preservatives. *See* Preservatives
Formaldehyde
  aspartame and, 50
  smoking and, 65
Fountain, Maggie Gillott, 44,
  99–100
Freedom, 9–10
Free-range chicken, 81
Freshwater, Amy, 259
Fructose
  as a sugar substitute, 73
  sugar use and, 69
Fruit juice sweeteners, 74
Fruits
  calcium in, 91
  constipation and lack of, 220
  eliminating pesticides by washing,
    57
  food combining and, 111, 113
  gas and, 219
  sulfites and, 54–55
Functional bowel disease, 224

Gallup polls, 83, 137

Gas, 218–220
  food allergies and, 239
  foods causing, 219
  frequency of, 218–219
  ways to avoid, 219–220
Gastritis, 220
Gastroesophageal reflux disease
  (GERD), 220
Gelman, Michael, 200
Genetics. *See* Heredity
Gifford, Kathie Lee, 200
Ginger, in cure for sprains, 255
Glucose, and sugar use, 68, 69, 70
Gluten, and food allergies, 238
Goals, and gusto, 166
Goldenseal, 254
Goodwin, Frederick K., 193
Grains, calcium in, 90
Growth hormones. *See also*
  Recombinant bovine growth
  hormone (rBGH)
  milk and, 86, 94–95
  sleep and, 149
Guacamole, recipe for, 288
Gulf War Syndrome, 50
Gusto (B.E.S.T. step 10), 8, 158–167
  being ready for, 160–161
  confidence and self-esteem and,
    164–165
  food and, 165–166
  imagery and visualization and,
    167
  looking good and feeling good
    and, 162–164
  makeover tips for wimps, 45
  setting goals and, 166
  "toy box" theory on, 161–162

Hahnemann, Samuel, 249
Harvard School of Public Health, 53
Hay, William, 107–108
Headache
  caffeine and, 61
  cure for, 254
Healing, and sleep, 150, 157
Healing crises, and detoxification,
  41–43

Health
  caffeine and risks to, 58–59, 63–64
  dairy use and, 84
  excuses for not being healthy, 12–13
  importance of, 39
  laughter and, 140
  Marilu Henner 101 on, 270
  milk and, 88
  overweight people and, 177, 182–183
  questions to think about, 13
  stress and, 135
Heartburn
  causes of, 227–228
  food allergies and, 239
  treating, 228
Heart disease
  dairy use and, 84, 88
  fat and, 123
  fiber and, 228, 229
  genetics and, 192–193
  high blood pressure and, 191
Heart rate, and exercise level, 128–129
Henner, Lorin, 110, 159
Hennings, Mary Ann, 101
Hepburn, Katharine, 166
Herbal supplements, 245, 251–253
Herbal tea, 71, 154
Herbs, 48
Heredity, 185–199
  Family Health History Chart and, 186, 188–189
  genes and diseases in, 190–228
  understanding implications of, 186–189
High blood pressure, 191–192
Hippocrates, 210, 251
Holmes, David S., 139
Homeopathic medicine, 249–251
Honey, as a sugar substitute, 73
Honey meringue frosting, recipe for, 301
Hormones. *See also* Growth hormones; Recombinant bovine growth hormone (rBGH)

protein and, 31
smoking and, 65
Hot dogs, 53
Human growth hormone (HGH), and sleep, 149
Hydrolyzed protein, 52
Hyperactivity, and sugar use, 77
Hypoglycemia, 76

Ice cream
  alternatives to, 103, 104
  fat and, 126
Imagery, 167
Imagine Foods, 102, 103
Immune system
  food allergies and, 238
  inflammatory bowel disease and, 225–226
  sleep and, 150
Inflammatory bowel disease (IBD), 225–227
  treatment of, 226–227
  types of, 226
Insomnia, 152–155
  depression and, 193
  solutions to, 153–155
  types of, 152–153
Institute of Medicine, 172
Insulin, and diabetes, 199, 230
International Agency for Research on Cancer, 51
Intolerances, food, 238–241
Iodine, 281
Iron, sources of, 281
Iron deficiency, and milk, 96
Iron supplements, 220
Irritable bowel disease (IBS)
  causes of, 224–225
  constipation and, 221
  fiber and, 229
  preventing, 225
Italian restaurant, ordering in, 263

Jet lag, cure for, 254
Jolt, 58
Josie's restaurant, 257
  ordering from the menu at, 262

recipes from, 283–305
Journal, 235–237
  bowel movements tracked in, 213, 242
  example of, 235
  exercise tracked in, 241
  food allergies and, 240
  food intake tracked in, 237
  menstrual cycle tracked in, 243
  reasons for keeping, 235
  sleep tracked in, 242–243
  weight tracked in, 236

Kidneys, and reading your face, 202–203
Kids. *See* Children
Kola nut, 62
Krank20, 58
Kushi, Michio, 201

Labels
  caffeine use and, 64
  food allergies and, 238, 240
  monosodium glutamate (MSG) disguised on, 51–52
  saccharin and, 71
  synthetic fats and, 53
Lacto-ovovegetarianism, 82
Lactose, 74
Lactose intolerance
  diarrhea and, 222
  gas and, 219
Lactovegetarianism, 82
Langdon, Harry, 162–163
Lanza, Louis, 102
  Josie's recipes and, 285–306
  on ordering in a restaurant, 257–258
  on stocking your pantry, 267–268
Laughter, 140
Laxatives, 221
La Leche League, 97
Lead, and detoxification, 41
Learning Deficit Disorder, and sugar use, 77
Lecithin, and cholesterol, 123–124
Legumes, calcium in, 90

Lessing, Doris, 39
Lifestyle
   food combining and, 106
   freedom and, 9–10
   identifying what is right in, 38–39
   interpreting symptoms and,
      234–235
   journal recording, 235
   making the commitment to
      change, 36–39
   Rainbow Theory of, 16–18
   unhealthy diet of Americans and,
      1–3
   yin and yang and, 19–22
Lip exfoliants, 206–207
Lipids, as a nutritional category, 33
Liquor. *See* Alcohol
Liver
   reading your face and, 203
   stool content and, 217
Low-fat diets, 178–180
Lunch, stocking your pantry for, 265
Lungs, and reading your face, 203
Lymphoma, and milk use, 97
Lysine, for cold sores, 253

Macadamia apple pie, recipe for, 305
Macrobiotics, 83, 272
Magnesium
   morning sickness and, 254
   sleep and, 156
   sources of, 281
Makeover tips for wimps, 45
Maltose, 73–74
Massage, 142, 143–144
Matoin, John, 110
Mattes, Richard, 178
Mayo Clinic, 173
Mayonnaise, alternatives to, 103
Meat (B.E.S.T. step 4), 5–6, 78–83
   makeover tips for wimps, 45
   naturalness of vegetarian diet and,
      79–80
   nonmeat sources of protein and,
      82–83
   organic meat and, 56
   slaughterhouse methods and, 80–82

sugar use and, 70
Meatless diet. *See also* Vegetarian diet
Meat loaf, vegetarian, recipe for, 296
Meat loaf sauce, vegetarian, recipe
   for, 297
Medications
   caffeine in, 62
   constipation from, 220
   dieting and, 172–173, 180–181
   sleep problems and, 154
Meditation, 245
Melatonin, 154–155
Melons, and food combining, 111,
   113
Menstrual cycle
   lifestyle journal on, 243
   listening to your body on,
      243–244
Meringue, honey frosing, recipe for,
   301
Metamucil, 229
Methanol, from aspartame, 50
Milk. *See also* Dairy (B.E.S.T. step 5);
   Lactose intolerance
   alternatives to, 101–102
   components of, 93
   how cows are treated and
      production of, 85–87
   irritable bowel disease and, 224
   lactose from, 74
   rBGH (recombinant bovine
      growth hormone) and, 54,
      94–95
Milton, John, 167
Minerals. *See also specific minerals*
   skin care and, 207–209
Miso, 104, 223
Miso broth with vegetables, recipe
   for, 283
Miso dip with mango, organic red,
   recipe for, 286
Moisturizers, 206–207
Molasses, 71
Monosaturated fats, 121–122
Monosodium glutamate (MSG),
   51–52
Mood

food use and, 234
sugar use and swings in, 76–77
Morning sickness, cure for, 254
Motion sickness, cure for, 255
Mouth
   digestion and, 211
   reading your face and, 202
MSG (monosodium glutamate),
   51–52
Mucosa, 210

Naps, 155
National Cancer Institute, 228
National Council for Health
   Statistics, 180
National Institute of Child Health
   and Human Development, 97
National Institutes of Health, 222
Natural remedies, for sleep
   problems, 154–155
Needles, in acupuncture, 248–249
Nervous system, and reading your
   face, 202
Neurotransmitters, and stress, 141
Niacine, 281
Nicotine. *See also* Smoking
   detoxification and, 41
Nitrates, 52–53
Nitrites, 52–53
No-fat diets, 178–180
Norepinephrine, and stress, 141
NutraSweet, 50, 72
Nutrients
   cholesterol and, 123–124
   dairy and deficiencies in, 96
Nutrition. *See also* Diet
   aspartame and, 72
   categories in, 31–33
Nuts
   food allergies and, 238
   food combining and, 114–115
   mood and, 234

Obesity
   diet and, 181–183
   genetics and, 191
Olestra, 53–54, 181

Oral hygiene, and sugar use, 76
Organic food, 55–57
  FDA definition of, 56
  fear of pesticides and use of, 57
  meat and, 56
  stocking your pantry, 268–269
Oriental Diagnosis, 201
Osteoporosis, 195–198
Ovarian cancer, and dairy, 95
Overweight people
  eating habits and, 169, 176–178
  heartburn and, 228
  heart disease and, 192–193
  obesity and, 181–183
  sugar use and, 76

Pantothenic acid, 281
Pantry, stocking, 264–268
Papain, 228
Papaya, 228
Parton, Dolly, 18
Pasta, organic artichoke flour, with
  organic plum tomato sauce,
  recipe for, 290
Peale, Norman Vincent, 164
Peptic ulcer, 220
Personality
  posture and, 33
  yin and yang and, 20
Pesticides, 57
Phenylketonuria (PKU), 50
Philbin, Regis, 200
Phospholipids, 33
Physiology, and yin and yang, 20
Phytochemicals, 281–282
Pico de gallo, recipe for, 299
Pie crust, healthier, recipe for, 304
Pilates, 127
Plant derivatives, and yin and yang,
  22–24
Plant foods, and yin and yang,
  22–24
Plant protein, 82
Plant protein extract, 52
PMS, cure for, 255
Polyunsaturated fats, 122
Portobello mushroom fajita, recipe
  for, 298

Posilac, 94–95
Posture, and balancing/centering
  your body, 33
Potassium, 282
Potentiatization, in homeopathic
  medicine, 250
Pregnancy, and caffeine use, 64
Preservatives. *See also* Chemicals
  (B.E.S.T. step 1)
  dangers of, 49–55
  detoxification and, 41
  reasons for using, 46–48
Protein
  examples of B.E.S.T. foods in, 34
  food combining and, 108–109,
    111, 112, 117, 118
  jet lag and, 254
  milk and, 93
  no-fat diets and, 179
  gas and, 219
  nonmeat sources of, 82–83
  as a nutritional category, 31
Pumpkin pie, healthier, recipe for, 303
Pure Food and Drug Act of 1906, 80

Qi, 245–246

Rainbow Theory, 16–18
Raw honey, 73
rBGH (recombinant bovine growth
  hormone)
  diary and, 94–95
  dangers of, 54
Recipes, 285–306
  apple-cranberry chutney, 293
  banana honey spice cake, 300
  black bean dumplings, 285
  butternut squash soup, 284–285
  chili-seared shrimp marinade, 287
  chopped vegetable salad, 289
  cilantro tofu sour cream, 299
  guacamole, 288
  healthier biscotti, 302
  healthier pie crust, recipe for, 304
  healthier pumpkin pie, 303
  honey meringue frosting, 301
  macadamia apple pie, recipe for,
    305

miso broth with vegetables, 283
organic artichoke flour pasta
  with organic plum tomato sauce,
  290
organic red miso dip with mango,
  286
pico de gallo, 299
portobello mushroom fajita, 298
stir fry sauce, 294
super soy Caesar, 291
sweet potato–red miso gravy, 297
teriyaki sauce, 295
turkey tortilla roll, 292
vegetarian meat loaf, 296
vinaigrette, 289
Recombinant bovine growth
  hormone (rBGH)
  diary and, 94–95
  dangers of, 54
Rectal cancer, and fiber, 230
Red Dye #2, 49
Red Dye #3, 49–50
Red meat. *See also* Meat (B.E.S.T.
  step 4)
  sugar use and, 70
Red miso dip with mango, organic,
  recipe for, 286
Refined white sugar, 68–69
Reich, Wilhelm, 245
Relaxation, 139, 245, 247
Reston, James, 246
Rice Dream, 99, 101, 103
Rice milk, 101
Rice syrup, 73
Rivers, Joan, 163

Saccharin
  dangers of, 54
  description of, 71
Salmonella, 82
Salt
  as a preservative, 48
  reading your face and eating, 199,
    202
Saturated fats, 98, 121
Seasonal Affective Disorder (SAD),
  194
Secondary amines, 52

Selenium
   skin care and, 208
   sources of, 282
Self-awareness, 247
Self-esteem, and gusto, 164–165
Selye, Hans, 134
Serotonin
   stress and, 141
   sugar use and, 77
Set point, and weight, 184
Shelton, Herbert M., 108
Shiatsu, 249
Shrimp marinade, chili-seared,
   recipe for, 287
Skin, 204–207
   collagen and, 204–205
   diet and, 204
   exfoliating, 206
   moisturizing, 206–207
   stress and, 207
   sun and, 205
   vitamins and minerals for,
      207–209
Skin brushing
   benefits of, 144–145
   face and, 146
   technique of, 145–146
Skin cancer, 208
Slaughterhouse methods, 80–82
Sleep (B.E.S.T. step 9), 8, 147–157
   brain and, 151–152
   constipation and, 221
   depression and, 193
   description of, 148–149
   immune system and, 150
   insomnia and, 152–155
   lifestyle journal recording, 235,
      242–243
   makeover tips for wimps, 45
   naps and, 155
   natural remedies for problems in,
      154–155
   need for, 147–148, 149–150
   sleep journal and, 155–157
   stages of, 149
Sleeping pills, 154
Sleep journal, 155–157
Small intestine, and digestion, 211, 212

Smith, Roger, 185
Smoking, 65–66
   caffeine and, 63
   chemicals in, 65
   heartburn and, 227
   heart disease and, 192
   osteoporosis and, 197
   psychological problems and, 65
   weight gain from quitting, 66
Snacks, stocking your pantry for,
   265–266
Soda. *See* Soft drinks
Sodium
   high blood pressure and, 192
   sources of, 282
Sodium nitrate, 52–53
Sodium nitrite, 52–53
Soft drinks
   caffeine in, 58, 59, 62
   gas and, 219
Soup, butternut squash, recipe for,
   284–285
Sour stomach, 227
Soybeans, and cholesterol, 123–124
Soy Caesar, Super, recipe for, 291
Soy milk, 99, 101–102, 104
Spastic colon, 224
Spices, 48
Sprains, cure for, 255
Starches
   as carbohydrates, 32
   food combining and, 108–109,
      111, 112, 118
   gas and, 219
Sterols, 33
Stevens, Lillie Kae, 69, 100, 214, 237
Stir fry sauce, recipe for, 294
Stomach, and digestive process,
   211–212
Stools. *See* Bowel movements
Stress. *See also* Exercise and stress
   (B.E.S.T. step 8)
   cold sores and, 253
   diarrhea and, 222, 223
   diet and, 247
   heart disease and, 193
   insomnia and, 153–154
   irritable bowel disease and, 224, 225

lifestyle journal recording, 236
   skin care and, 207
Stress management, and quitting
   smoking, 66
Stretching, and exercise, 130
Stroke, 191, 229
Substance P, 207
Sucrose, 73
Sugar (B.E.S.T. step 3), 5, 67–71
   as carbohydrates, 32
   chemically processed, 75
   children and, 67–68
   constipation from, 220
   effects of using, 68–69
   impact on body of, 76–77
   kicking the habit, 69–71
   makeover tips for wimps, 45
   naturally processed, 75
   reading your face and eating, 202
   stress and, 141
   taste changes and, 70–71
Sugar crash, 77, 141
Sugar substitutes
   dangers of, 50–51
   description of, 71–74
   diarrhea and, 222
Sulfites
   dangers of, 54–55
   as a preservative, 48
Sun, and skin care, 205
Sunscreen, 206
Sunette, 49, 72
Surge, 58
Sweeteners
   artificial. *See* Sugar substitutes
   chemically processed, 75
   naturally processed, 75
Sweet One, 49, 72
Sweet potato–red miso gravy, recipe
   for, 297
Synthetic dyes, dangers of, 49–50

Tahini, 104
Tai chi, 245
Taste
   changing your palate and, 27–29
   chewing and, 29–30
   sugar use and, 70–71

Tea, caffeine in, 59, 62
Teriyaki sauce, recipe for, 295
Textured vegetable protein (TVP), 52
T.G.I.Friday's restaurant, 259, 261
Thyroid cancer, and artificial colorings, 50
Tofu, 104
  as an egg alternative, 102
Tooth decay, 76
Toothpaste, fluoride, 76
Toxins
  cleansing, 40–43
  fiber and, 229
  skin care and, 206
"Toy box" theory on gusto, 161–162
Transit time, in bowel movements, 215
Travel, and diarrhea, 223
Triglyceride fats, 33
Turkey, organic, 56
Turkey tortilla roll, recipe for, 292

Ulcerative colitis, 226
Unsaturated fatty acids, 282
Urgent diarrhea, 223

Veganism, 82
Vegetables
  calcium in, 89–90
  constipation and lack of, 220
  eliminating pesticides by washing, 57
  food allergies and, 239
  food combining and, 111, 112
  sulfites and, 54–55
Vegetable salad, chopped, recipe for, 289
Vegetarian diet, 105
  naturalness of, 79–80
  nonmeat sources of protein and, 82–83
  ordering in a restaurant and, 257–258
  reasons for using, 83
Vegetarianism, types of, 82
Vegetarian meat loaf, recipe for, 296

Vegetarian meat loaf sauce, recipe for, 297
Vinaigrette, recipe for, 289
Viral infection
  diarrhea and, 222
  inflammatory bowel disease and, 225
Visualization, 167
Vital energy, 245–246
Vitamin A, 207, 277
Vitamin B1, 277–278
Vitamin B2, 278
Vitamin B3, 278
Vitamin B6, 278
Vitamin B12, 278
Vitamin C
  cholesterol and, 123–124
  skin care and, 208
  sources of, 279
  vegetarian diet and, 83
Vitamin D
  milk and, 89
  osteoporosis and, 198
  sources of, 280
Vitamin E
  cholesterol and, 123–124
  vegetarian diet and, 83
  sources of, 280
Vitamin K, 281
Vitamins. *See also* Antioxidants
  fat and, 120
  herbal supplements and, 252
  milk and, 93
  skin care and, 207–209
  sleep and, 156
  sources of, 277–281
  synthetic fats and, 53
  vegetarian diet and, 83
Vita-Soy, 101
Vitiello, Michael, 148

Water
  examples of B.E.S.T. foods in, 34
  food combining and, 116, 117
  in milk, 93
Weight
  ideal, 183

lifestyle journal recording, 235, 236
  set point and, 184
  vegetarian diet and, 83
Weight gain
  eating habits and, 169
  heart disease and, 192–193
  quitting smoking and, 66
  sugar use and, 76
Weight loss
  eating habits and, 169
  exercise and, 127–128
  fiber and, 230
  food combining and, 106
  ideal weight and, 183
  not using dairy products and, 98–99
  vegetarian diet and, 83
Welland, Christal, 100
West, Mae, 163
Wheat bran, 229
Withdrawal symptoms, from caffeine, 61
Witter, Terry, 123
Wolf, Jacqueline, 225, 226
World Health Organization, 51
Wrinkles
  face care and, 206
  reading your face and, 203–204

Yellow Dye #5, 50
Yin and yang
  description of, 19–22
  extreme foods and, 22–24
  food and behavior and, 26–27
  headaches and, 254
  laughter and, 140
  personality and physiology and, 20
  qi in alternative medicine and, 245–246
  reading your face and, 201–204
  stress and, 142
Yoga, 245

Zinc, 282